UNDERSTANDING AND TREATING YOUR MIGRAINE

PAULA GREENSPAN

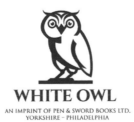

WHITE OWL

AN IMPRINT OF PEN & SWORD BOOKS LTD.
YORKSHIRE – PHILADELPHIA

First published in Great Britain in 2018 by
White Owl
An imprint of
Pen & Sword Books Ltd
Yorkshire - Philadelphia

ISBN 9781526725844

A CIP catalogue record for this book is available from the British Library.

Typeset in India by Vman Infotech Private Limited

Printed and bound in Malta by Gutenberg Press Ltd.

Pen & Sword Books Ltd incorporates the Imprints of Pen & Sword Books Archaeology, Atlas, Aviation, Battleground, Discovery, Family History, History, Maritime, Military, Naval, Politics, Railways, Select, Transport, True Crime, Fiction, Frontline Books, Leo Cooper, Praetorian Press, Seaforth Publishing, Wharncliffe and White Owl.

For a complete list of Pen & Sword titles please contact

PEN & SWORD BOOKS LIMITED
47 Church Street, Barnsley, South Yorkshire, S70 2AS, England
E-mail: enquiries@pen-and-sword.co.uk
Website: www.pen-and-sword.co.uk

or

PEN AND SWORD BOOKS
1950 Lawrence Rd, Havertown, PA 19083, USA
E-mail: Uspen-and-sword@casematepublishers.com
Website: www.penandswordbooks.com

For Andy, Lane and Zack
my biggest motivation for staying balanced

CONTENTS

ACKNOWLEDGEMENTS

This book wouldn't exist if it weren't for Kate Bohdanowicz, who had faith in my idea and pitched it to the publisher. Speaking of whom, Lori Jones, Janet Brookes, Kate Bamforth, Emily Robinson, and everyone at White Owl, have been absolutely wonderful. They must be the loveliest book publishers on Earth.

I'm also very grateful to my editor, Carol Trow, for her kind words, encouragement and expertise.

A massive thank you to all of the experts who gave up their time to be interviewed, and the people who live with migraines who allowed me to tell their stories.

Finally, I'm very lucky to have super-supportive family and friends, especially Andy, Lauren, James, Debs, Jenny and Lisa, who never seem to tire of listening to me talk about migraines. Or if they do, they don't show it!

INTRODUCTION

In the course of writing this book, I've spoken to a lot of people about their migraines. One thing that stands out for me is the stories that they told me about the one migraine they'll never forget. For some people it was their first migraine, for others it was one that made them miss a friend's wedding or came on right in the middle of a holiday and ruined it for them. But the one thing that connects them all is that these migraines always stopped the people who were having them in their tracks and made them realise the sheer power that migraines can have over your life.

With that in mind, I thought I'd share my own migraine story. For me, that defining moment in my experience with this disorder was when I got a migraine with aura at a toddler group with my not-quite 2-year-old son. I'd taken him into the loo to change his nappy when I found myself blinking over and over because my vision wasn't entirely clear. At the time, I didn't understand my migraines well enough to realise that this was a sign that I had to act – fast – to keep things from spiralling out of control. Instead, I buried my head in the sand and hoped my fuzzy vision didn't mean that I was about to get a migraine. What I didn't know then, was that pretending a migraine isn't happening is like pretending a tornado isn't heading your way. That storm is going to hit whether you like it or not. So you can carry on with what you're doing and get whacked with the full force of it, or you can do whatever it takes to minimise the impact. Because if you're not prepared, it can be devastating.

On that day at the toddler group, I finished the nappy change and took my little boy back out to the echoey hall full of bright lights and squealing toddlers. Which, let's face it, is the last place you want to be when a migraine starts. As I tried to watch my little boy happily clambering down a plastic slide, I realised with cold fear that part of my vision had become pixelated, and other bits of my sight were just not there. For me, this was a typical aura. I'd get a blurry crescent on either one side or the other (it could change from attack to attack, and even move during a single aura) and the rest of my vision would look as if someone had found an old jigsaw with some bits missing and had forced the pieces together anyway, meaning that everything in front of me looked a bit like a knock-off Picasso. Needless to say, my eyesight was useless. In minutes, I found myself sitting on the floor, staring blankly into the space in front of me, not able to focus on the group of children racing about just inches away.

Thankfully, I wasn't alone at the toddler group. A friend, Vicky, asked if I was OK and when I told her that I was having a migraine, she was pretty sympathetic. Which was lucky, really, because not everyone is that kind about them. I, on the other hand, felt like a drama queen causing a fuss in the middle of a sea of babies who needed attention.

After all, I wasn't broken or bleeding. I wasn't even in any pain. Yet.

What I hadn't realised was that I was at the start of one of my worst migraines to date, and that I was beginning to feel confused and disengaged from what was going on around me, like I was experiencing the world from inside a perspex box. It meant that I also couldn't think clearly to help myself. Or look after my son.

Vicky, on the other hand, was an absolute angel. She asked if there was anything she could do and when I said I wished I had a Diet Coke because the caffeine helps ease the aura, she immediately got me a cup of tea. It was an obvious solution, really; the lovely ladies who ran the toddler group were making cups of tea for the parents anyway. But by that point, I was so befuddled that the idea hadn't even occurred to me,

Within minutes of drinking the tea, the aura started to dissipate, almost fizzing before my eyes like a bubbly glass of Alka-Seltzer. The only trouble was that as the aura cleared, the pain crept in. It was a sharp, searing pain in my head that slowly grew and grew like a balloon expanding. When I could finally see again, I grabbed my moment and got my son in the pushchair, then headed straight to the chemist for paracetamol and ibuprofen, swallowing them dry before starting our 15-minute walk home.

Thank goodness I decided to stop for those painkillers, because by the time we were halfway home, the pain was so bad that my knuckles had gone white from gripping the pushchair handle in agony. My son seemed none the wiser and, somehow, I managed to get him inside and down for his nap before I collapsed into bed myself.

By the time we both woke two hours on, my migraine hadn't cleared, but the pain was at a more bearable level. I carried on walking around in that perspex box for three days, though, alternating paracetamol and ibuprofen so I could cope until it went away and I could finally think clearly.

And once I felt like myself again, I decided that this couldn't go on.

In my case, this doozy of an attack made me realise that this disorder was something I had to start taking more seriously – for my own sake and for the sake of my family. There had been days when it had stopped me from working, evenings when I'd missed out on nights out with friends, and times when I generally walked around in a moody daze, just trying to get through it.

The thing was, while sleep, caffeine and painkillers helped, once a migraine started, nothing would actually put a stop to it, I just had to wait for it to come to its natural end. I was fed up of riding it out time after time, and I'd had enough of fearing my next attack. It was time to stop hoping that it wouldn't happen again and start finding ways to prevent my migraines altogether, or, at the very least, make them less severe. It was time to take control.

I've been living with migraines since I was a teenager, although for years I just thought they were PMT headaches. In fact, I used to call them: 'my headaches that don't go away,' because although at that stage paracetamol or ibuprofen would help, the pain would always come back. And I knew it would always go on like this for three days, so I just kept taking painkillers until it finally ended.

Over the years, my migraines got worse and worse. My GP eventually prescribed a migraine medication called Sumitriptan and while the medication could sometimes stop or delay a migraine, I hated the side-effects. The drug made me feel like I was having an odd out of body experience, which was actually worse than the perspex box feeling that a migraine left me with. Add in the fact that the medication didn't always work for my migraines, and that meant that I sometimes ended up dealing with the migraine symptoms and the side-effects all at once. So I decided that I'd rather find a way to cope with my migraines on their own than take my chances with the side-effects as well. To put it plainly, I decided to stick with the devil I knew.

Without Sumitriptan, I considered trying a stronger painkiller, but a chat with the chemist told me that many of the stronger ones available could make me sleepy. I knew I couldn't take the painkillers and look after young children at the same time, so that left me with good old ibuprofen and paracetamol.

But, really, that left me with virtually no protection against the migraine tornado. If my only defence against it was regular-strength painkillers, I had no doubt that I was going to get flattened. In the past, going for acupuncture and osteopathy had been good for my migraines. But there's no cure for migraines in either conventional or alternative medicine, and if I didn't keep up regular appointments, the effects of these treatments wore off quickly. At £50 a pop, that could get pretty pricey and I wondered if there was a way to feel well without shelling out all that cash.

Don't get me wrong, I think alternative therapies are fantastic. I'd support anyone who found something that helped keep their migraines at bay, and I'd encourage you to follow the advice in this book alongside anything else you're doing that works for you. Having said that, what you're going to read here is the result of my research into ways of preventing migraines without spending loads of money. Then if you want to do more on top, go for it. Do what it takes and do what works for you.

So what works for me? Acupuncture and osteopathy, although (touch wood) I don't need either at the moment. Instead, getting enough good quality sleep, switching to decaf coffee, staying hydrated, avoiding lactose, eating regularly throughout the day and doing yoga most mornings keeps me balanced enough to avoid sticky situations at toddler groups. Sounds pretty simple, doesn't it? That's because it can be.

The tricky bit is that what works for me might not work for you. Migraines are a very individual experience. How I feel during a migraine and what brings on my attacks might be very different to your symptoms and triggers.

It sounds pretty isolating, doesn't it? It can certainly feel that way when you're lying alone in a dark room in the throes of an attack, too. That's why I've interviewed people who get migraines, so you can read their stories throughout this book. Although the details of each person's experience is different, there are things that unite us all. As you're reading the stories, you'll probably read symptoms that sound familiar and treatment options that you can relate to. You might even pick up a few ideas for dealing with migraines that could help with your own attacks, too.

What you won't read in this book is a one-size fits all solution for preventing migraines. Believe me, if there were a magical way to cut migraines out of all of our lives, I'd be singing it from the rooftops. Unfortunately, this disorder just doesn't work that way.

So what does that leave us with? Small, easy lifestyle choices that can make a real difference. What choices you need to make in your day-to-day life to help with your migraines will be individual to you but as you read on, and, hopefully, begin to keep your own migraine diary, what's triggering your migraines will become clearer and what changes you could make for the better will too. As you carry on reading you'll see that many of the lifestyle choices you can make to improve your migraines are great on their own, but also work in harmony with one another. For example, by simply getting the sleep you need, you can eliminate a common trigger. Staying fit will help with your migraines as a standalone lifestyle choice too. But on top of all the good you'll be doing by sleeping well and keeping in shape, doing the right exercise for you will also help you to sleep better. Lots of these little things that you can do to manage your migraines will work to support each other. Which will only help you to feel better in the long run.

And please, if you're on any sort of medication or have any other health conditions or concerns, speak to your doctor before changing your lifestyle, so he or she can help you to choose what's best for you.

As well as speaking to people who get migraines, I've also interviewed migraine specialists, doctors, health and wellbeing experts – and even my sister, a counselling psychologist who uses mindfulness with her clients and teaches it to other therapists – to get advice on the lifestyle changes that could help ease and prevent your migraines.

Finally, you might have heard experts use the word 'migraineurs' to describe people who get migraines. You won't read that word again in this book, because I don't want to be defined or labelled by my migraines and I don't want you to think that way either. While it's true that you can't wish away your migraines – and believe me, I've tried – I refuse to lie back and think, 'I'm a migraineur, that means I'm going to suffer.'

We're all human and sometimes I'll do something that I shouldn't, or something will happen in my life that's out of my control, and the result is that I'll have a migraine. That's OK, because I know that most of the time I'm doing the right things to keep my body balanced. That means that if I do happen to get the odd migraine, it won't be as severe as it once might've been. Plus, I'm completely prepared to deal with it now and I know exactly what to do to get through it.

Yes, I get migraines, but I'm not going to let them get me.

PART ONE

THE BASICS

'Migraine stops everything.'
Lauren, 42

Chapter One

GETTING INSIDE YOUR HEAD: GET TO KNOW YOUR MIGRAINES

'A migraine is different to a normal headache. When I get a migraine, I feel so disconnected from what's going on around me, it's like I've got a bucket on my head. It stops me from functioning.'

Julia, 37

What is a Migraine?

That's a good question. If you asked five different people who live with migraines, you'd probably get five different answers. Why? Because the way it feels when you get a migraine is different for everyone.

From the time when you sense your first early warning symptoms starting, right through to that magical moment when you realise that you're finally feeling better, the experience that you have during an attack won't be the same as anyone else's. Sure, there are things that you'll have in common with other people you know who have migraines, for example, you and your mum might both feel sick when you've got one. But that doesn't mean your migraines are just like your mum's. It might be that you feel better after a long sleep, while your mum might need to take soluble painkillers and lie still in a dark room. That's because just as there's no one way to get a migraine, there's also no one way to prevent or treat them. While that makes migraines tricky to manage, the good news is that it means there will be lots of things that you can try.

Researchers used to think migraine was a vascular condition, which means that it's related to the blood vessels. This is because there are changes to your blood flow and your blood vessels when you have an attack. But thankfully, research into migraines is ongoing, and even though these vascular changes do take place, experts now believe that blood vessels aren't the root of the problem. Migraine is now considered to be a neurological disorder, which means that it's related to the nervous system, although unfortunately at this stage nobody knows what causes you to get migraines and there's no test that you can have to get diagnosed.

If you can't be tested for migraines, how does your doctor know you're getting them? By asking you about your experience with them. When you have a migraine, you'll get a collection of certain symptoms in a certain order. The symptoms might vary a bit from person to person and even from one of your attacks to another, but keeping track of what you're feeling when you get a migraine will reveal a pattern. And, as you'll find as you read on, that pattern isn't just useful for diagnosing your migraines, but also when preventing and treating them, too.

Some of these symptoms are pretty unusual. The migraine sufferers who were interviewed for this book often said, 'This might sound strange, but...' when describing what their attacks were like. Yet, to another person who gets them, experiencing odd sensations during a migraine is something that happens all too often. Even if they're saying that they see weird flashing lights before their eyes, and you get such a sore jaw that you feel like your teeth are falling out, you're still dealing with the same disorder. Your symptoms don't have to be the same to get comfort from knowing you're not alone.

So, migraines are a bit of a mystery, and to top it off, there's no cure. Frustrating, right? Don't worry. You don't need to know why you suffer from migraines in order to understand how to reduce the number of attacks that you get or to even avoid them altogether. As everyone's migraines are different, the aim of this book is to help *you* to figure out the best way to prevent *your* migraines. If you read something that doesn't apply to you, ignore it, and just make the most of the advice that does work for you.

So, What *Do* We Know About Migraines?

'Migraine is a genetic condition that means you have a low threshold for responding to triggers,' says Dr Fayyaz Ahmed, Consultant Neurologist with an interest in headache at Royal Hull Infirmary.

It's a complex disorder that experts are still trying to fully understand, but it's thought that a migraine starts with some abnormal activity in your brain which can affect things like blood vessels and nerve signals. Experts believe that chemicals in the body like serotonin and hormones like estrogen can play a part, too.

'Fundamentally, migraine is a disorder of sensory processing,' explains Peter J. Goadsby, Director NIHR/Wellcome Trust King's Clinical Research

Facility and Professor of Neurology, King's College London. 'Migraine sufferers are often sensitive to light, but they're not getting extra light. It's the perception that light is unpleasant.'

How does this happen? There are two competing theories about what happens when you're exposed to something that you're sensitive to, like the light that Professor Goadsby was talking about. One is that something in your brain generates a pain signal. So, if you have a glaring light shone in your eyes, somewhere in your brain a pain signal goes off. But that pain signal wouldn't go off in the brain of someone who doesn't get migraines. The other theory is that normal signals are fired in your brain in response to the light, but those signals are somehow misinterpreted as pain signals when you have a migraine.

Either way, what matters to you is that the bright light hurts. A lot. And that it's because you have reactions to triggers like that light that other people simply don't. We'll talk more about triggers later on, but they're basically the things that are harmless for most people, but for you, they can set a migraine into motion. So, while your friends might be able to douse themselves in perfume without so much as a niggle, or your husband can drink a massive cup of strong coffee first thing every morning without a worry, you may find these things can trigger migraines.

Anyone can get migraines – men, women, even some children – but according to the World Health Organisation, women are twice as likely to suffer from migraines, and this is probably because the natural fluctuations of a woman's hormones can be a trigger. There's a whole chapter dedicated to hormones later on, which will be helpful if you think your migraines are connected to your periods or to the menopause.

While anyone can get them, migraines are probably genetic. This means that your parents or grandparents are likely to have had a history of headaches, even if they weren't diagnosed with migraines. In fact, Dr Ahmed says that only half of migraine sufferers ever get a diagnosis. This might be because their migraines have been misdiagnosed as something else, or it might be because they're not severe enough to need help from the doctor, although, chances are, if simply popping a paracetamol were enough to stop your migraines, you wouldn't be reading this right now. You probably already know that while some attacks may be less severe than others, migraines can be debilitating. In fact, migraine was found to be the sixth most disabling condition in the Global Burden of Disease study done by the World Health Organisation. Often a bad migraine can be like an ink stain that seeps into every area of your life and leaves its mark.

Professor Goadsby says: 'Migraine doesn't shorten life, it robs you of time.'

That's so very true. When you have a migraine, you might not be able to work, spend time with your family or have any sort of social life. You've probably cancelled plans or called babysitters in at the last minute when a migraine has left you unable to carry on as you normally would. And it can be pretty frustrating to have to do that over and over again.

It's difficult to say how often that's likely to happen because the frequency of your migraines is as unique as you are. If you're lucky, you might only get a few in your lifetime, but on average, people who get migraines have them one to three times a month. That's a lot of migraines over the course of a year, let alone in a lifetime.

One thing's for sure, you're not alone. According to the charity Migraine Action, one in every seven people in the UK suffers from migraines. The Migraine Trust says that there are over 190,000 migraines happening every day in the UK. That's a lot of people struggling with this disorder each and every day.

Still, just because migraines are common doesn't mean that you have to let them win. Even if your entire family has migraines, and you've had more sick days than you can count thanks to your disorder, you can still take control of it. The first step is to try to understand your own experience. Then you'll be in a good position to figure out how to reduce the number of attacks you have, make them less severe, or even stop them altogether.

Migraines and Children

According to The Migraine Trust, only about 10 per cent of children get migraines. When a child has a migraine, it can be a bit different to an adult migraine. They can have shorter attacks, affecting their whole head rather than just one side, and sometimes the sickness is worse than the headache. In some cases, a child can have stomach pain but no headache at all, which is called an abdominal migraine. Children with migraines can also get dizzy and feel sensitive to light and noise. Although they're less likely to experience the visual disturbance of an aura, if a child does get one, it's likely to come on at the same time as the pain, rather than before it, like an adult's migraine. As children grow and change, their migraines change with them. If they've had abdominal migraines, their symptoms might become more like typical migraines as they get older. But it's also reassuring to know that some children with migraines will grow out of them, too.

My Migraines
Julia, 37

'My migraines began when I started university at 18. I put myself under a lot of pressure at the time and whenever I'd take a break and try to have some fun in the student bar, I'd get a migraine.

'It's the same whenever I'm working hard now. I'm a youth theatre director and I tend to work in bursts of intense long hours. I know that once the busy period stops, I'll get an attack.

'I'm sensitive to the weather as well, so I'm likely to get several migraines at the start of each season.

'For me, a migraine usually starts with a manic feeling, where I rush around, full of energy. After that, the pain sets in. I get pain in my face that's so bad my face feels solid, like a mask. I usually feel sick or dizzy and need to lie down with a cold cloth on my head, too.

'I try to drink lots of water and take painkillers as soon as I feel a migraine coming on, but I've never thought about trying to do things to prevent them altogether. If I could do that, it would be amazing!'

Chapter Two

THE STAGES OF A MIGRAINE

'I've learned that when I feel extremely tired in the evening, I'm going to wake up with a migraine the next day.'

Linda, 68

Why Do You Need to Understand the Stages of Your Migraines?

By now, you probably get that no two migraines are exactly the same. Yet, even though what you experience may be a bit different each time, you'll still go through the same four – sometimes five – stages of migraines. Knowing what these stages are, and how they tend to feel for you, can help you to get a better understanding of what you're going through. And understanding your migraines is the first step to preventing them.

In order to identify the stages of your migraines, you need to keep track of them in some way, such as using the migraine diary sheet that you'll find later on in this book. The aim of this is to identify patterns in how you feel during your attacks. Unfortunately, this means that you have to have a few migraines before you can see that pattern developing. While nobody wants that, the sad truth is that those migraines are going to happen whether or not you keep track of them. And, if you do take note of what you're going through in the different stages of your migraines, you'll be able to recognise your symptoms from the start. Then you can react more quickly when you feel a migraine coming on and take steps to prevent it from getting worse. Plus, at some point, hopefully you'll even be able to prevent attacks, too. So, you're playing the long game but it'll be worth it in the end.

What Are the Different Stages of Migraines?

Stage One: The Warning Phase

You might also hear the warning phase called the premonitory phase – like a premonition. It's also known as migraine prodrome, which means an early sign or symptom. Whatever you call it, this phase can last from one hour to two days. It's a sneaky phase though, and it can be so subtle that you might not even realise it's happening, or you may even mistake your warning symptoms for something else. For example, let's say one Saturday morning you feel absolutely bursting with energy. Maybe you're feeling so full of beans that you decide to go out for a run. While you're bounding around the block feeling fantastic, a migraine will be the last thing on your mind, won't it? But this energetic surge can actually be a warning symptom. The trouble is, at that moment when you're bouncing around like Tigger, you're hardly going to be thinking, 'This is awful, by tomorrow I'll be lying in a dark room feeling sick.'

Fast-forward a few hours to the point when you're in the full throes of your migraine, and you're likely to be feeling a lot less lively. However, if you take note of how you've been feeling – even before the worst of the attack hit – and the same thing happens in a month's time, you'll have a chance of recognising that this energetic feeling can be a warning sign of a migraine. Then you'll be in a position to do something about it straight away.

And you should react quickly to your warning symptoms, too. If you've been prescribed migraine medication, this is when you need to take it. That said, even at this early stage, you can't just pop a pill and expect it to do all the hard work. Once you know – or even suspect – that you might be barrelling head-on into a migraine, that's your cue to take care of yourself. Make healthy food choices and drink lots of water. Cancel your plans to go to spinning class or out for drinks with your friends and have an early night instead. Spotting your early warning signs and taking action now, whether you're taking tablets, drinking water or getting some sleep, may actually prevent the next – more severe – stages of your migraine from developing. If not, it could still make the symptoms less severe. And wouldn't that be nice?

Common Warning Phase Symptoms

- Irritability
- Mood changes
- Energy bursts
- Extreme fatigue
- Food cravings
- Increased thirst
- Nausea or appetite changes
- Muscle pain
- Aphasia – temporary trouble with words
- Concentration problems
- Increased urination
- Digestive problems
- Sensitivity to sound or light
- Yawning or trouble sleeping

My Migraines
Linda, 68

'I had my first migraine at 12 years old. I didn't have another one until after I'd had my youngest child when I was 26, and from then on they happened almost weekly. It took a while for me to learn the warning signs, but I became aware of an acute tiredness some evenings, and then I'd wake up with a migraine the next day. I eventually realised that this tiredness was a part of my migraines and now I take Migraleve when that starts rather than waiting for the pain and nausea to kick in. Although, at times, it's been so bad that I've had to take a prescription medication called Zomig. Fortunately, often after a good night's sleep, I feel much better, although my head still feels a bit muzzy afterwards. I get migraines much less frequently now, but I always carry Migraleve with me so I can take it as soon as I feel the early symptoms starting. That's my way of coping.'

Stage Two: Aura

The aura stage of a migraine can be pretty scary, especially if you haven't spotted any warning phase symptoms beforehand. One minute, you're going about your day as usual, the next, you're seeing flashing lights or have blind spots in front of your eyes. Although most of us think about the aura as something that disturbs your vision, you could have other symptoms, too, like dizziness or feeling weak.

What's more, according to a study done at the Montefiore Headache Center in New York, a very small number of people – around 0.7 per cent of people with migraines – think that they're smelling something that isn't actually there when they're experiencing a migraine aura. This is called olfactory hallucination and if you get it, you might smell burning or smoky odours, rubbish, sewage, or, if you're lucky, something nice like coffee.

Not everyone who gets migraines will have an aura, but the good news is that if you do, the aura doesn't last very long. You'll probably only have it for less than an hour. The bad news is that once the aura's gone, it's a sign that you could be moving on to the painful and disabling attack phase next.

That said, you might find that you just get the aura and don't experience any pain afterwards. This is called a silent migraine. While it might sound like a dream to anyone who suffers with the full-on agony of a painful attack, it's still a migraine and it can still be very frightening and debilitating.

- seeing flashing lights, coloured spots, stars or zig zags
- blind spots or temporary blindness
- tunnel vision
- dizziness
- vertigo
- numbness
- tingling
- pins and needles
- weakness on one side
- hallucination – seeing, hearing or smelling things that aren't there, like seeing bright lights or smelling coffee
- trouble speaking

My Migraines
Simon, 43

'My migraines start with an odd, withdrawn feeling. Then the aura always kicks in and for me it looks like the effect you're left with after looking at a naked light – like a flashbulb in my eye. Then this changes again, and it's like there's a wavy line through the middle of my vision, as if half of what I'm looking at is under water, and I can't focus. The aura can last for up to 40 minutes and I haven't been able to find any way to relieve or shorten this phase. I've tried sitting in a darkened room and I've even worn eye patches but they haven't worked. So I've learned that I just have to weather it out.

'Thankfully, I've never had an aura while I've been driving, but I've had migraines come on when I've been out, or at work. It can be quite debilitating, and it's tricky, especially when I have to explain to people who I don't know very well, or who've never had a migraine, that there's a reason why I've suddenly become quiet and isolated.

'After the aura clears, I get pain on one side of my head. Although I've tried different medications, nothing stops a migraine once it starts. I actually find that munching on things, like salt and vinegar crisps, or chewing on a big wad of chewing gum to really get my jaws working helps to relieve the pain.

'I once had a migraine come on in the night that was so bad, I felt like my head was exploding. My partner took me to A&E, and as my speech was slurred, the doctors thought I'd taken something.'

Stage Three: The Attack

When it comes to the most intense stage of a migraine, the word 'attack' doesn't quite cut it, does it? People who've been interviewed for this book have described their migraines as: 'intense', 'debilitating', 'crushing pain', and 'like being stabbed in the brain', which is a much more accurate description of what it's like to live with this disorder. Still, the third stage of a migraine is called the attack, and it's kind of the main event. If nothing else, this is the stage that most people who don't get migraines associate with the condition. It's the time when you'll get bone-crushing pain, nausea or vomiting that lasts for up to three days and can literally bring you to your knees.

Chances are, if you suffer from migraines, the attack phase is the bit that you find the most painful and debilitating, and it's also the part of your condition that you'd most like to avoid. Also, once the attack phase hits, it's a lot harder to treat your symptoms, which means that from this point onwards it can feel like you're at the mercy of your migraine, desperately trying to do anything you can think of to ease the pain and sickness while you wait for it to pass. This is why it's much better to try to prevent migraines if you can, or to act fast and get treatment as early into the migraine as possible, certainly before the attack phase hits. If you do that you have a chance of having a less severe attack – or putting a stop to the migraine altogether before you even reach the attack. Early treatment is even more important if you tend to be sick during the attack stage, because once you start vomiting it will be harder to get the medication you need into your system.

Attack Phase Symptoms

- Throbbing pain, often on one side of your head or at the front of your head
- Pressure in the head
- Stomach pain
- Nausea and vomiting
- Sensitivity to light, sound, smell and touch

> **Can't Touch This**
>
> When you get a migraine, your senses can be heightened so much that it actually becomes painful. The name for this type of migraine symptom is allodynia, and it's when something causes you pain even though it shouldn't. So perfectly normal things like brushing your hair, for example, going out in the sunshine, or even resting your head on your pillow, could actually hurt while you're in the throes of an attack. Allodynia can be tricky to treat, even with painkillers, which is another reason why it's important to catch a migraine before this sort of symptom sets in.

Stage Four: The Resolution Phase

The resolution phase is that wonderful time when the worst of your migraine eases. You might be one of the lucky people who finds that your attacks stop very quickly, for example, you might be sick and suddenly feel better afterwards, or if you're able to get a couple of hours' sleep, you may wake up and realise that the pain is gone. And while that's possible, unfortunately most of the time, a migraine won't disappear that quickly. Usually, once an attack gets its claws into you, it can take its time to slowly slip away.

Stage Five: The Recovery Phase

So, the throbbing pain in your head has finally eased off and you've stopped being sick. You should feel on top of the world now, right? Wrong. Migraines are fierce little suckers and they really do leave you reeling afterwards. Welcome to the recovery phase.

The recovery phase of migraines is also called the postdrome phase. Postdrome is just another word for the symptoms that you get after an attack has passed. Lots of people call it a migraine hangover and for the day or so that you're in this phase, it really does feel like you're recovering from a big night out. Only you've had a lot less fun getting to this point.

Just like during a hangover, right now you could be dehydrated, especially if you've just spent a couple of days barely eating and being sick. So be kind to yourself. You might find that you're as hungry as a bear coming out of hibernation, so eat well to help your body to find some balance again. Drink lots of water, too. And although you might be fed up of the sight of your bedroom walls by now, get some rest. It's called the recovery phase for a reason so take the time to allow yourself to recover.

Recovery Stage Symptoms

- Fatigue
- Confusion
- Mood changes
- Lack of concentration
- Stiff neck

Types of Migraine

In the third edition of their *International Classification of Headache Disorders,* The International Headache Society has classified different types of migraine to help doctors to diagnose and treat them. You'll probably recognise at least one of them, because it's possible for one person to get more than one type of migraine. They include:

- **Migraine with Aura**

This is one of the two major types of migraine and it's exactly what it sounds like – a migraine where you experience an aura before the attack stage. You might get a headache during the attack, or you might have other symptoms of a migraine and aura, but no pain.

- **Migraine Without Aura**

The other major type of migraine is one that you get without the aura. You could get symptoms like pulsing pain – probably on one side of your head – nausea and sickness, and it may be easier to lie still because it could feel worse when you're moving around.

- **Migraine with Brainstem Aura**

With this type of migraine, you might have an aura but you'll also get other symptoms like tinnitus, which is hearing things like buzzing or ringing in your ears, vertigo, which is when you feel like you're spinning, fainting and slurred speech.

- **Hemiplegic Migraine**

Hemiplegic migraines can be pretty scary. They're like a normal migraine with aura, but with other additional symptoms like pins and needles and weakness on one side. If you have hemiplegic migraines, there's a fifty per cent chance that your children will, too. When it runs in families it's called familial hemiplegic migraine.

- **Retinal Migraine**

If you have retinal migraines, you get visual disturbances. But these migraines are different to migraines with aura because with a retinal migraine you get these effects, like flashing lights, or loss of vision, in just one eye. The disturbance tends to last up to an hour and you'll usually get it in the same eye each time.

- **Chronic Migraine**

People who get chronic migraines have attacks almost relentlessly. The criteria doctors use to diagnose chronic migraines are pretty specific. If your migraines are chronic, it means you have headaches on 15 days of the month for at least three months, and you'll have migraine symptoms for at least eight days of the month. Migraines with or without aura can be chronic.

If you have chronic migraines, they can have a massive impact on your life. Your ability to work, have a social life, keep up with hobbies and housework can all be affected by your migraines. To put it bluntly, they're disabling.

One thing to keep in mind when you're dealing with chronic migraines is that it becomes easy to overuse medications, simply by taking them too often to try to manage your attacks. Only, this can actually make your condition worse. If you're concerned about medication overuse, ask your GP or specialist for help.

My Migraines
Natasha, 35

'I'd never had any type of migraine until I had my first hemiplegic migraine seven months ago. I had just arrived home after a five-day holiday in Turkey and my partner Stu and I had driven for two hours from the airport before stopping at a rest stop. I was just standing there, when suddenly it felt like the room was spinning. Stu helped me to sit down and got me some water, but I was so dizzy that I couldn't even drink it. The next thing I knew, I felt a shooting pain go up the back of my neck and my right hand started going tingly and feeling numb. Then I got pins and needles in my right leg and I realised that I couldn't move it. It was absolutely terrifying. Stu phoned 999 and by the time the paramedics arrived I was so out of it that although I could hear them, I couldn't respond. They thought I was having a stroke and took me to hospital where scans showed that it wasn't a stroke but instead they suggested it was a hemiplegic migraine. The paralysis lasted for about 18 hours but I still couldn't walk properly for two days.

'I had two more of these migraines over the next couple of months. Once Stu thought I'd fallen asleep because I was lying down, but I felt like I'd been drugged and I couldn't open my eyes or move.

'I don't know what my triggers are yet and although I love to travel, it's made me frightened of flying. Last month I flew to Germany and I didn't have an attack, but I didn't relax and have a few drinks like I normally would, either, because I was afraid it would trigger another migraine.'

Chapter Three

TRIGGER HAPPY: WHAT IS A MIGRAINE TRIGGER?

'I fear my migraines because they can be so debilitating. But I've figured out a few things that can trigger them, like not eating and drinking enough when I'm busy, and I get them less often now.'

Lauren, 42

What is a Migraine Trigger?

Migraine triggers are things that you come across in your regular day-to-day life to which you have a sensitivity and can lead you to have a migraine.

What this means is that somehow normal, harmless things that your body senses, like bright sunlight or the strong smell of coffee brewing, affects you in a way that ends up in a migraine. And the things that cause you to react in this way – such as the sunlight and the smell of coffee – are called your triggers.

This probably sounds pretty familiar and you may have already had some success in finding out what some of your triggers are. After all, it sounds pretty obvious. If you get a migraine after drinking wine, then alcohol is a trigger for you, isn't it? Possibly, but you might also find that you can have some wine one day and feel absolutely fine, while on others, a single glass tips you over the edge.

That's the funny thing about migraine triggers, they're not as clear-cut as you might think. While you might have some major triggers that you learn you absolutely have to avoid, being exposed to a single trigger isn't always like a massive bullet with 'migraine' written down the side heading straight for you. And it generally won't be just one thing that flips a switch to send you spiralling head-first into an attack.

Triggers can often work in combination with one another, and, when they're piled one on top of the other, can set off an attack. So you might find that, on a good day when everything else is in balance, you can have that glass of wine. Only if you happen to be overtired and standing outside on a bright sunny day, the drink will be the last straw.

Imagine you have a massive vice hovering around your head, ready to squeeze at any time. As a migraine sufferer, that probably isn't too difficult to picture! Each time you expose yourself to a trigger, that vice is cranked, bringing it closer and closer until you finally feel the pressure on your skull. So, often a single trigger puts you more at risk of a migraine than you'd be without it and if you add trigger on top of trigger, eventually that vice is going to tighten to the point where a migraine is inevitable. It's a group effort, on behalf of your triggers.

The point at which you tip over the edge and your triggers cause a migraine is called your migraine threshold. So it might be that lack of sleep cranks that vice several times over and crosses your migraine threshold every time. Or, you might have had the odd glass of wine after work during a stressful week, and that might have been fine for a while. Only, when the sky suddenly erupted into a thunderstorm, the change of weather was too much on top of everything else and tipped you over and past your threshold.

Whatever your triggers are – and don't worry if you don't know any of them yet because we'll talk about that a lot later on – keep in mind that it can also take up to eight hours for a trigger to cause a migraine. So whatever you were doing immediately before your warning symptoms started might not be what actually triggered them in the first place.

All of this is probably making triggers sound like something terrifying that you'd rather hide from, but actually, getting to know your triggers is really important. Because the great thing about them is that they don't just make your migraines happen, they can be the key to preventing them, too.

In order to free yourself from the squeeze of that vice, you've got to figure out what causes it to tighten. Just like everyone's migraines are different, everyone's triggers vary, too, although there are some common ones that are more likely to be giving you trouble.

In order to figure out what your triggers are, you have to identify a pattern with your migraines. Let's say that you go to bed late one night and develop a migraine the following day. And maybe you notice that this happens on another couple of days when you've had less sleep than usual. It's likely that lack of sleep could be a trigger for you– particularly as this is a common trigger.

Yes, this does mean that you have to have a few migraines before you can spot the patterns and confidently do something to prevent them, but those migraines were going to happen anyway, right? You might as well use them to put together some information that can help you to feel better in the long run. Keep in mind that migraines like to keep you on your toes and you might have to reassess your triggers from time to time, too.

'Migraine evolves and triggers vary over time,' says Professor Goadsby. 'What might not trigger you one day will trigger you in a month's time.'

Some Common Migraine Triggers

Just like the title says, this is a list of some of the more common migraine triggers. You might find that you're absolutely fine with some – or all – of these things and that it's actually something completely different that triggers your migraines. But when you're thinking about what your triggers might be, this is a good place to start. We're going to look at some of them in more detail later on.

- Sleep – both too much and not enough
- Stress
- Certain food and drinks such as alcohol or processed meats
- Hormones
- Visual stimulation like bright lights or screen use
- Hunger or dehydration
- Intense exercise
- The Pill
- Tension in your jaw
- Strong smells
- Changes in weather or seasons

Balance is Everything

When it comes to migraines, balance means keeping things on an even keel. Anything that takes your body to too much of an extreme will put you off balance and make you vulnerable to an attack. This balance is about avoiding crazy ups and downs and not shocking your body with things like overtiredness and massive hangovers. You might need to make little – and sometimes not-so-little – lifestyle choices that can have a huge impact. For example, eating regularly, staying hydrated or making sure you get the right amount of sleep can all help to create the regularity that you need. And, just like triggers, these lifestyle choices will be different for everyone. So, the first step is to learn what your body needs to stay balanced.

It's time to get selfish here, because getting control of *your* migraines is all about you. While there are eight million other people out there in the UK getting migraines, none of them will be exactly like you and none of their migraines, their triggers, or the steps they need to take to keep those triggers balanced, will be exactly like yours either.

So let's say you've worked out a few of your triggers. In an ideal world you'd be able to find your balance by avoiding those triggers completely and live happily ever after without ever having a migraine again. Only, like everything else with migraines, it's not always that simple, because some triggers are easier to avoid than others. For example, if drinking alcohol is a trigger for you, then staying teetotal will help you to prevent migraines. Easy. However, if getting too much sleep can trigger your migraines, you need to know how much sleep is right for you, what time is best for you to go to bed and get up in the morning, and how to get the best quality sleep during that time. These are all things that you can figure out, you just need to know how to approach it.

Even once you've worked all of this out, life can tip you off-balance a bit. No matter how committed you are to preventing your migraines, there's also no way to guarantee that you won't ever get stuck in traffic when your stomach's rumbling at lunchtime, or that you'll never catch a whiff of someone's extra-strong perfume ever again. But don't worry. Even though the thought of getting a migraine can be terrifying, you don't have to stop living in order to avoid them. The trick is to keep that balanced lifestyle most of the time. This will put you in the best possible position to deal with those accidental triggers, and hopefully even avoid the full force of a migraine attack when you do become faced with them.

The goal here is to stop feeling like you're endlessly spiralling from migraine to migraine with little life in between. Instead, you should actually be able to live your life, and enjoy it, without spending all of your time, money and energy trying to stay migraine free.

The next section of this book will take you through some common migraine triggers and explain how to figure out which ones affect you, and what lifestyle choices you can make to find the balance you need. Understanding this will help when you're using your migraine diary, which you'll read a lot about in this book. Your migraine diary comes up so much when we're talking about preventing migraines because this diary is the most important tool you've got. When you're ready, you can use the diary for keeping note of your lifestyle and your migraines in order to help you track down your triggers, and eventually find some balance. If a paper diary doesn't appeal, you might want to try an app, like Migraine Buddy, which does the job, too. Whatever you use, what matters is that you consistently keep track of what's going on with your migraines. As you do and as you start to remove triggers from your lifestyle, you'll begin to free yourself from the shackles of your migraines.

My Migraines
Lauren, 42

> *'I remember my first migraine really clearly. I was 22 and it was one of the worst ones I've ever had. I'd just started my master's degree in political journalism and it was the first week of that course, so it was a bit of a stressful time because I was trying to do new things and make friends on my course. I went to a meeting of the university newspaper with a girl I'd just met, but while we were there I developed this awful headache and started to feel sick. I felt so ill that I had to leave early. To make matters worse, I couldn't get on the bus to go home because I was afraid I'd be sick on the bus. So instead I struggled through an hour-long walk home and cancelled my plans for the evening. Little did I know, it was the first of many times that I'd have to cancel plans at the last minute. I had no idea what had caused me to feel so unwell, but my mum had migraines and when I told her what had happened, she suggested that I might have them too.*
>
> *'From then on, I got a migraine every month with my period like clockwork. Sometimes I'd wake up with it and think: 'Oh God, I've got the migraine headache,' because by that point, there was nothing I could do about it. I spoke to my doctor who took me off of the low estrogen pill I'd been taking and swapped it to a different one, which did help a bit. I was also given Paramax, a soluble medication that's a combination of paracetamol and an anti-sickness medication. Taking Paramax as soon as I felt the headache start would stop me from vomiting, although I'd still feel sick. Without it, I'd be sick all day, like an awful stomach bug, and spend the rest of the time curled up in a ball with my eyes closed. And even once that had passed, I'd spend a day with a fuzzy head, feeling like somebody's trampolining in my brain.*
>
> *'Over the years, I learned that not eating and drinking enough can trigger migraines, so I make sure I eat little and often and drink enough*

water. Stress can be a trigger, too, and I wouldn't dare drink a glass of red wine, now.

'When I get a migraine, I have to spend at least a day in bed because there's nothing that I can do but have the migraine. I've even missed out on two weddings I'd been invited to because of my migraines.

'I'm not on any form of hormonal contraception now and I only get migraines every six months or so. Although I'm dreading menopause because I'm afraid my migraines will come back with a vengeance. If they do, I'll try anything to prevent them. They're so debilitating.'

PART TWO

PREVENTION

'If you have a healthy lifestyle, you eliminate a lot of triggers.'
Dr Fayyaz Ahmed, Consultant Neurologist with an interest in headache

Chapter Four

SLEEP

'I haven't slept for more than eight hours a night in months, because I know that sleeping for too long increases my risk of getting a migraine.'

Karen, 52

What's the Connection Between Sleep and Migraines?

That's a good question. You probably don't need to be told that sleep is an important issue for people who live with migraines. For some people, there are times during an attack when nothing will do but a good snooze. Tiredness can be a symptom of migraines, particularly during the warning and recovery phases, so take advantage of it and sleep if you can. You might also find that a bit of shut eye can relieve your symptoms or even stop a migraine in its tracks.

Having said that, there's a chance that you're sitting there reading this in complete disbelief after suffering through migraine after migraine that have kept you wide awake all day and night. That's because when you live with migraines, sleep can be a bit of a chicken and egg issue. You might find that sleeping badly can cause you to get migraines, or that your migraines can cause you to sleep badly. Which is all pretty exhausting, really.

'The areas of the brain involved in migraine are intimately connected with the areas involved with sleep,' says Professor Goadsby. 'It's clear the mechanisms are inter-linked.'

So sleep and migraines are connected, but experts don't actually know why they're so tightly woven together. What does this all mean for you? If you want to avoid migraines, you need to get a good night's sleep – every night.

What Happens When You're Sleeping?

Before we dive into tips for more restful nights, we need to understand a bit about sleep itself. There are two different types of sleep, rapid eye movement

(REM) sleep and non-rapid eye movement (NREM) sleep. During an average night, you move back and forth through NREM and REM sleep around four or five times, and each time is called a sleep cycle.

NREM sleep has three stages: Stage 1, when you're drifting off; Stage 2, when you're in a light sleep; and Stage 3, when you're sleeping heavily. If you have a sleep disorder, like night terrors or sleep walking, that will come into play during Stage 3. Incidentally, people who live with migraines are more likely to have these sorts of sleep disorders.

Back to your sleep cycles. About 90 minutes after you fall asleep, you'll then go into your first stage of REM sleep. In REM sleep, the only parts of your body that move are the muscles you use to breathe and your eyes, which rapidly dart back and forth. This is the time during the night when you have most of your dreams, too. Your first period of REM sleep will last for about 10 minutes and they'll get longer over the course of the night, up to around 90 minutes.

How to Work Out the Best Sleep Patterns for You

So, you know that you need to get a good night's sleep in order to prevent your migraines, and the next step is to figure out what that actually means for you. You see, everyone has a circadian rhythm, which is like an internal body clock, and yours might not be the same as your friend's or partner's. That's why some people are naturally up at the crack of dawn while others are night owls. The trouble is, between screen time, family and work demands – and of course, migraines – keeping you awake, it's easy to get out of sync with your natural body clock. If you're not in tune with your body clock, you probably never feel properly rested. Of course, not getting enough rest can then be a trigger for another migraine, which will make you feel even more tired. You can see how this can easily turn into a vicious cycle, which needs to be put right.

It might seem like the answer is to simply get more sleep, or to try to make up for any lost sleep by napping or sleeping longer at the weekend. Yet for some people, this 'extra' sleep can actually be a migraine trigger, and you might be doing yourself more harm than good. What you need to do instead is learn how to understand your own personal body clock and get the proper sleep that *you* need.

So How Much Sleep Should You Get?

The National Sleep Foundation in the US did a study and they found that most adults need between seven and nine hours of sleep a night. Keep in mind that this is just an average, though, which means that there are people who will need more or less sleep, as well. Those of us who feel refreshed after fewer than six hours a night are called 'short sleepers,' while 'long sleepers' need at least ten hours a night.

If you've regularly been getting less sleep than you need, chances are you're feeling pretty tired – and then some. You could be irritable, you might have trouble concentrating and you may find that you have poor judgement, too. On top of that, when you consistently get too little sleep you can end up with something called a sleep debt, which puts you at risk of health conditions like diabetes, heart disease and obesity.

Oversleeping can make you feel pretty sluggish, too, even if you're just trying to make up for a bad night's sleep by lying in. And, of course, being off-kilter by getting the wrong amount of sleep, whether it's too much or not enough, can leave you more likely to get a migraine.

Fortunately, even if you haven't been getting the sleep that you need for some time, you can still get things back on track. Assuming, that is, that you don't have a medical problem that's disrupting your sleep. For example, sleep apnoea, which is when you stop breathing for at least ten seconds at a time while you're sleeping, and this interrupts your sleep. Depression is another condition that can affect your sleep, although in this case it can cause you to oversleep. Those aren't the sort of sleep issues that we're talking about here and they require a bit more support to sort out. If you think a medical problem is interfering with your sleep, it's best that you ask your GP for help.

So how do you work out how much sleep you should be getting each night? Sleep Coach Rachel McGuinness suggests giving yourself a week to do it. 'The best way to understand how much sleep you need is to go to bed when you initially feel tired and wake up naturally,' she says. 'Try this for a week when there is nothing in your diary, and you will find out exactly how much sleep your body needs.'

The idea is to take a week to prioritise your sleep, which is worth doing if it's triggering migraines. Over the course of this week, keep note of how much sleep you're getting each night and as the days go on, you'll notice a pattern emerging that will show you how much sleep you need. Even better, try to think of your sleep in terms of the number of 90-minute sleep cycles you should be getting rather than in one massive chunk of time. So, if you find that you naturally sleep for nine hours a night, you're aiming for six sleep cycles. It might sound slightly more complicated but there's a good reason for doing it this way. It's because you'll feel at your best if you wake up when you're in a light sleep stage. Think about it, have you ever been jolted awake from a really deep sleep and felt woozy, groggy and heavy? If you wake from the wrong part of your sleep cycle every morning, you're going to start every day like that. And if you feel rubbish morning after morning, you're more likely to have migraines.

Timing is Important, Too

Once you've taken note of your sleep for a week, you'll know how many sleep cycles you're aiming for each night. But if you want to feel rested, you shouldn't get these sleep cycles at any random time during the day. The time that you go to bed and the time that you get up make a difference, too. This is because the circadian rhythm in your body, which is governed by a little area in your brain called the hypothalamus, runs on a 24-hour clock. In order to maintain the rhythm, you should be sleeping during the same few hours of those 24, each and every day.

Pay attention here because this is an important bit – this means that you should be going to bed and getting up at around the same time every day. Sure, life gets in the way and it might not be realistic to expect your head to hit the pillow at, say, 10pm every single night. But aiming to do this, whether it's a Tuesday when you've got to get up early for work the next day, or a Saturday when you can have a lazy day off, will help you to keep things on an even keel, and, of course, eliminates a migraine trigger, too.

'Our brain loves consistency and routine, it doesn't understand holidays or weekends,' says Rachel. 'If we go to bed late and get up late on our days off or on holiday, it puts our body clock out of kilter and technically into a different time zone. When we have to go to bed earlier or get up earlier for work again, we feel tired during the day. This is known as social jet lag.'

Does that mean you can never lie in on a day off? Rachel says that if you struggle to sleep, you could probably give yourself an extra 30 minutes in bed. Again, this is individual, and you might be able to sleep in for as long as an hour, but gauge how you feel after you wake up. If you try it once and it backfires, don't do it again. It's as simple as that.

In order to keep your sleep consistent, you need to know what time you should be getting to sleep each night. Your ideal bedtime actually depends on what time you need to get up in the mornings. Nobody knows that better than you. After all, whether you've got to get up for work or to take the kids to school in the morning, you know what time you have to set your alarm for, right? All you have to do is set it on your days off, too – allowing for as much leeway as you can handle, if you choose to – and stick to it. Then count backwards from your wake-up time for the number of sleep cycles you need each night, and, bingo, there's your bedtime.

For example, Let's say you need those six 90-minute sleep cycles each night, which add up to nine hours in total. If your alarm goes off at 6.30am, you'll want to be in bed and ready to sleep by 10.30pm. Even better, once you've got used to it, chances are you'll start waking up naturally at around the time of your alarm anyway. That's a good sign that you've really cracked it.

How to Get Better Quality Sleep

We've talked about quantity, now let's look at the quality of your sleep. It's all well and good that you're spending the right number of hours in bed, but it's only when you wake up feeling properly rested that you're getting the kind of sleep you need to avoid triggering a migraine. And the great thing is, that feeling will last throughout the day, too. It might seem like trying to get good quality sleep is as easy as grabbing a fistful of smoke, but most of us can do it if you have what experts call good sleep hygiene. While the term 'sleep hygiene' sounds like advice to take a bath before bed (and, by the way, this can help), it's actually about the good habits that you can adopt to help you to get a better night's sleep.

These habits are small changes that you can make, which all add up to a more peaceful night:

- **No Screen Time Before Bed**

  The first easy step towards better quality sleep is to avoid screen time for at least half an hour before you go to bed. That includes TV, tablets, phones and computers. Why? They mess with your body clock. There's a hormone in your brain called melatonin, which controls your circadian rhythm. Melatonin production is naturally suppressed by blue light waves that come from the sun, which means that being in daylight keeps you awake. If you go outside in daylight, your body produces less melatonin and that helps it to know that it's time to be awake. Then as the sun sets in the evening and daylight dims, melatonin levels rise, helping you to drift off. Those blue light waves that keep you awake come from the lights in screens, too. So if you look at a screen at bedtime, you're exposing yourself to blue light waves. That light can confuse your body and hold back the melatonin production that helps you to fall asleep.

  In order to stop this from happening, shut off your screens a minimum of half an hour before bedtime. Or if you're really serious about it you could go as far as keeping technology out of the bedroom to help create the best atmosphere for sleep.

  That said, there may be some leeway. 'E-readers are fine,' says Rachel. 'As long as the screen is turned right down to reduce the glare.'

Some e-readers, like the Kindle Fire, have a mode to reduce the blue light waves. Don't feel that you have to rush out and buy one, but if you have an e-reader with this feature, try it.

Otherwise making it a habit to watch telly, check Facebook or play video games earlier on in the evening and then snuggling up with a good book before bedtime could seriously help you to drift off.

- **Create a Cosy Atmosphere**

Do your curtains let in light? Is the room a touch warm? Can you hear trains whooshing past nearby? These are all things that you need to consider. Everything about the conditions you're sleeping in, from the softness of your sheets to the lumps in your mattress, is important. Take some time to think about what might be keeping you awake at night because simple little things like getting blackout blinds, keeping the room between 16 and 21 degrees, and using ear plugs if it's noisy, can make a big difference to the quality of your sleep.

- **Get Some Exercise**

According to a poll done by the National Sleep Foundation in the US, people who exercise are more likely to say they've had a good night's sleep than people who don't. You're playing the long game here because it can take four months of regular exercise to have a positive impact on your sleep. Still, if that helps to keep your migraines at bay, it'll be worth it. We'll talk more about how exercise can help migraines a bit later on, but when it comes to your sleep, the important thing is to do it regularly and be patient.

- **Have a Warm Bath Before Bed**

A shower will do too, but not a cold one. It's all about your body temperature, which naturally cools down throughout the afternoon. Like the daylight dimming, this cooling off tells your body clock that it's getting close to bedtime. So by taking a warm bath, you're giving your body a chance to cool down afterwards, sending a signal to your circadian rhythm that it'll be time to sleep soon. Just make sure that you get in the tub around two hours before your bedtime so you're not too toasty by the time you're tucked up in bed.

- **Don't Take Naps**

Or, if you really need a nap, then at least keep it short. Napping's another thing that's quite individual and you're really the only one who can tell if it will affect your overall sleep and how rested you feel throughout the day when you have a nap.

'As with anything it's about how you feel when you wake up and whether or not it affects your ability to get to sleep at night,' Rachel says. 'A short nap of 20-30 minutes can be beneficial and give you an energy boost. When it becomes a habit because you're not sleeping well, it could be interfering with your night time sleep.'

So if you've been relying on naps to get through the day because your nights are restless, it can start to backfire. In that case you might want to try skipping the naps to see if it helps.

- **Watch What You Eat and Drink Before Bed**

We've all been there, tossing and turning with indigestion after a heavy evening meal, or getting up and down in the night like a yo-yo because you need the loo after downing a glass of water before bed. When you think about it, what you eat and drink can have a massive impact on your sleep, and there's a lot that you can do to improve on it.

There are certain foods that can disrupt a night's sleep, like anything too fatty, acidic, or spicy and, of course, caffeine. Your morning coffee is called that for a reason, because it makes you feel more awake. For the best night's sleep, try avoiding caffeine after lunchtime.

If caffeine wakes you up, certainly alcohol can put you to sleep, right? It might seem like the answer to any sleep problem is to knock yourself out with a few glasses of wine. Yes, alcohol can help you to drift off more quickly, however, as alcohol affects the quality of your sleep, it's not going to make you feel rested the next morning. If you've been drinking, you're likely to have less of that all-important REM sleep and wake up earlier in the morning.

So what should you eat and drink before bed? Nothing heavy because if your digestive system is doing too much hard work, it can leave you tossing and turning. Instead, a light bedtime snack which contains the amino acid tryptophan is a good idea. Tryptophan is good for sleep because it boosts your melatonin levels, and you'll find it in foods like milk, hummus, nuts and seeds, bananas and oats. Rachel recommends snacking on something like hummus with a couple of oatcakes or a small bowl of porridge with half a banana 30-60 minutes before you go to bed.

Also, just like you wouldn't go to bed on a full stomach, you won't be able to sleep with a full bladder either. Try not to drink too much liquid in the two hours before bed so you don't have the disruption of getting up to go to the loo in the night.

- **Don't Smoke**

  Researchers at the University of Florida found that smokers lose 1.2 minutes of sleep for every cigarette smoked. Which is no surprise, because nicotine's a stimulant like caffeine. If you smoke, you're likely to have more trouble getting to sleep, get less sleep each night and have poorer quality sleep. Quitting will help, although you're likely to sleep better if you've never smoked at all.

- **Try Breathing Techniques**

  Once you're tucked up in bed, Rachel recommends giving belly breathing a go. 'Belly breathing calms down the stress response, stimulating the parasympathetic nervous system and helping the body relax,' she says.

  What's belly breathing? Well, of course, you don't actually breathe into your belly – that's impossible. When you're doing belly breathing, what you're trying to do is fill your lungs completely, instead of taking shallow breaths that only use the top of your lungs. The way to do that is to breathe deep enough so that your belly goes up and down with each breath. Hence the name, belly breathing.

  To do this type of breathing, lie down in bed, breathe in slowly through your nose and count one. Then breathe out slowly through your mouth and count two. Continue, counting all the way up to 10, and keep repeating until you fall asleep.

Sleep Disruption Beyond Your Control

Now, let's be realistic. While it's important for you to make consistent sleep a priority, life sometimes gets in the way and when that happens it can knock your sleep patterns out of whack. You might work shifts, have young children who are up in the night, or go on an amazing holiday that means you'll end up getting jet lag. So what do you do when things get off track?

First of all, do what you can to keep consistent, particularly if you're a shift worker and you have to go to bed at different times of the day. That means having a bedtime routine, such as taking a warm bath, then having a small snack, and snuggling up in bed with a book. If you follow this routine, whatever time you happen to go to bed, it will tell your body that it's time to sleep. When you find yourself heading home in the morning following a night shift, try wearing dark glasses to minimise the sun's effect on your sleep.

When it comes to jet lag, the trick is to try to adjust to the new time zone as soon as possible, which means as soon as you get on the flight. Rachel suggests changing the time on your watch once you've boarded the plane and bringing your own food along so you can eat meals according to the new time zone, rather than waiting for the airline to serve it on their schedule. If you're flying west, get out in the daylight as much as you can once you arrive. If you're flying east, staying indoors or keeping sunglasses on until the afternoon will help you to adjust. And if you really need it, take a 20-30 minute nap – but no longer so you don't risk disrupting your sleep the following night.

Does Better Sleep Really Mean Fewer Migraines?

Researchers at the University of North Carolina, Chapel Hill, did a study with 43 women who were living with something called transformed migraine. Transformed migraine is when you start off having the occasional migraine, but over time you get them more and more often until your migraines become chronic. The researchers gave 23 of the women instructions on how to improve their sleep, and they gave the others false instructions as a placebo. After six weeks, the first group had found their migraines were 29 per cent less frequent and 40 per cent less intense, while the other group had no change. The researchers then also gave the second group the proper instructions and after another six weeks, 43.6 per cent of both groups still had occasional migraines but no longer had chronic migraines.

My Migraines
Karen, 52

> 'Sleep is very important to me because I've noticed that if I sleep for too long each night I get a migraine. I have a FitBit that monitors my sleep and I strive for eight hours a night, but not too much more, because I know that 10 hours' sleep will trigger a migraine. I've found that going to bed and getting up at the same time each day helps, too.
>
> 'Hormones are another trigger for me. My migraines began when I was about 17 and first went on the Pill. A year later, I had a migraine that was so severely painful, and made me so sick, that I was scared I was having a brain haemorrhage and my partner rushed me to hospital.
>
> 'I found that avoiding hormone-based contraception helped to reduce the number of migraines that I was getting and the ones I did get were less severe. But they did get worse again when I started going through the menopause.

'My doctor has prescribed Rizatriptan. When I get a migraine, it usually starts with pain behind my right eye when I wake up in the morning. If I take Rizatriptan when I wake up in pain it can stop the headache, although I still get other symptoms. The only trouble is that the medication makes me feel really woozy and spaced out, which is pretty unpleasant. I know that I should take my tablet as soon as I realise I'm having a migraine, but I tend to kid myself that it's not happening and take it later than I should because I don't like the side-effects of the drug.

'I know the medication works, and I have acupuncture to help keep attacks at bay, too. I also try to exercise regularly and limit the amount of alcohol I drink, because I've realised that both of those things can help as well.'

Chapter Five

YOUR HORMONES

'My migraines are hormone related and I know I'll get one either the week before or the week after my period.'

Amy, 34

Migraines affect three times more women than men, and women's hormones have a lot to do with that. According to the Migraine Trust, around half of women who live with migraines say they're directly affected by their menstrual cycle. Why is that? Women's hormones fluctuate throughout each cycle and throughout different stages of their lives, too. And migraine sufferers can be sensitive to these rises and dips in hormone levels.

So this is one thing that really does divide the sexes. 'Men's migraines aren't affected by hormones,' says Dr Ahmed. It's as simple as that. But without wanting to exclude anyone, this trigger is such a big issue for women that it does need to be looked at more closely. And as this entire chapter is dedicated to the effect that women's hormones have on their migraines, if you're a man, feel free to look away now. Even better, skip ahead to the next chapter.

If you're a woman who finds that hormones are a trigger, you might have had your first migraine around the same time as your first period, or you might get them every month like clockwork. There are so many different things that happen throughout your life which can affect your hormone levels, and these things can also have an impact on your migraines. For example, you might find that pregnancy, going through menopause and taking the Pill can trigger your migraines. It's not all bad news, though. Changes in hormone levels can also have positive effects on some women and those same things might reduce the number of attacks you get, too. Like many things with migraines, there's no one blueprint to follow.

Menstrual Migraines

As well as migraines which are triggered by hormones, there's also a type of migraine called a menstrual migraine which affects less than ten per cent of women. If you get menstrual migraines, it will either happen in the two days before your period or the first three days after it starts. The difference between menstrual migraines and other types of migraines that get triggered by hormones is that menstrual migraines will only ever happen during these days. So you'll never get a migraine at any other time of the month. If you're not sure which type you get, keeping track of your migraines and your period in a diary for at least three months should help. With menstrual migraines you're also unlikely to have any aura.

'The drop in oestrogen is responsible for menstrual migraine,' says Dr Ahmed. If this all sounds very familiar, your doctor may be able to offer oestrogen supplements during the week before your period to level things out, or use hormone-based contraception to stop your periods, both of which can help with your migraines.

Your Period

According to the Migraine Research Foundation, 23 per cent of girls have had a migraine by the age of 17, compared with just eight per cent of boys. And this is probably due to the hormonal changes that teenage girls go through.

Your hormones will naturally fluctuate throughout your menstrual cycle, and although you didn't know it at the time, this started even before you got your first period. But, like any highs and lows, this hormone fluctuation can leave someone who lives with migraines feeling pretty off-kilter. Because of course, when your body isn't balanced, migraines can happen.

Researchers at the University of Cincinnati College of Medicine and Cincinnati Children's Hospital Medical Center did a study looking into the effect of the hormone progesterone on migraines in girls. They found that girls aged 8-11 were more likely to get a migraine when their progesterone levels were high, but from the age of 16 that actually reverses, and participants were more likely to get migraines if they had low progesterone levels. So this shows that as girls who live with migraines mature, their hormonal triggers can change, too.

After puberty, the ups and downs of a woman's hormones will usually follow a similar pattern each month or so. Just before your period starts each month there's a drop in the hormone oestrogen and this drop in oestrogen can also be a big migraine trigger for women.

Migraines and the Pill

Everything we've seen so far shows that as a woman who lives with migraines, you can be pretty sensitive to the hormones that naturally occur in your body. When you take the Pill, or other hormone-based contraceptives, you're introducing additional hormones into your body that wouldn't have been there otherwise, and this can have an effect on your migraines, too. You might even find that these extra hormones can balance things out, and that being on the Pill can help to prevent your migraines.

'If your GP will work with you on it,' says Ashley Grossman, Professor of Endocrinology at the University of Oxford, 'you can get the Pill prescribed for migraines. A low oestrogen pill can help with hormonal migraines, particularly those that come from the sudden fall of oestrogen before your period. The steady level of oestrogen may actually be helpful with migraines.'

That said, there are different types of Pill that you can take, and they might not all have this amazing effect on you. There's also a chance that going on the Pill at all could make your migraines worse, or you may need to try more than one Pill before you discover which one works for you. So if you haven't taken the Pill before, or you want to try to change which one you're taking, it's important that you talk to your doctor about your migraines first.

If you've found that taking the Pill can trigger your migraines, it may be because of the way it's taken. When your doctor prescribes the Pill, you'll either be given packs containing 21 or 28 tablets. If you've got 21, you'll have seven days out of each month when you don't take any at all. If you have 28, the last seven will be 'dummy' pills which don't contain any hormones. It's during this last week of each pack when you'll get your period. It doesn't matter which type of pack you have, if you take the Pill in a traditional way, you won't be getting any extra hormones into your body over those last seven days and you'll still have that oestrogen withdrawal which can trigger migraines.

Don't worry; if you find that this is a problem for you, there are still other options. You could talk to your doctor about taking the Pill continuously without a break, and you can do this safely as long as you do have a break every three to six months. When you do this, as you continue to get a dose of hormones for that entire time, you won't have a period over those months, which is safe, too. Another option is trying a progesterone-only pill, which doesn't contain any oestrogen. Or you could talk to your doctor about other types of hormone-based contraception, like the implant or injection, which are progesterone-only as well.

It's important to know that if you get migraine with aura, you should avoid certain types of Pill because it could increase your risk of having a stroke. This is why you should always talk to your doctor about migraines when you're discussing the Pill or speak to your GP if you're already on it and you've had an aura for the first time. She should be able to help you find out which Pill is best for you if you want to take it, although some women who live with migraines prefer to avoid all hormone-based contraception altogether.

Pregnancy

If your hormones have an impact on your migraines, then it makes sense that things might change for you during pregnancy, too. You may find that pregnancy is a time of blissful relief from attacks, but unfortunately, there's also the chance that they can get worse during these months.

In early pregnancy, oestrogen levels shoot up, and they can stay high until you give birth. So once your hormones settle after the first three months, you might find that you sail through the next two trimesters without a single migraine. Your levels of endorphins – which are hormones that act as natural painkillers – will be high during this time, too. This is great, because if you do happen to get a migraine during your pregnancy, you might find that they're actually less painful thanks to your high endorphin levels.

So. There you are, enjoying your blissful migraine-free pregnancy. Those months without migraines are an amazing break from attacks, but at some point, you're going to have the baby. And when you do, are your oestrogen levels going to come down with a bump? Possibly. Unfortunately, the flip side of the heavenly months of high oestrogen levels during pregnancy is that migraines can come back as your oestrogen levels drop once you've given birth. This drop can happen more slowly if you breastfeed, which is one reason why your periods aren't likely to return straight away. If you are breastfeeding, it may also help to keep migraines at bay until after your little one is weaned.

One thing that you've got to keep in mind is that there are other conditions that women can get during pregnancy that can cause headaches, vomiting, sensitivity to bright lights and visual disturbances, like pre-eclampsia, which can be dangerous for both you and your baby. If you get any sort of headache-related symptoms that concern you during your pregnancy, please call your doctor or midwife. Also, if you take migraine medication you should talk to your doctor about whether you can continue taking it during your pregnancy and afterwards if you're breastfeeding, too.

Menopause

You might think of menopause as the time when your periods stop. Of course, they do stop eventually, but it doesn't happen quite that suddenly. Rather than your body pulling the handbrake on your hormones out of the blue, the process of going through menopause can actually take years. In fact, there is a period of time before your periods stop for good called perimenopause, which can make you more vulnerable to migraines.

The average age for going through menopause is 51, but it could happen much earlier or later. And on average, perimenopause lasts for four years, but for some women it can take as long as ten years. During this time your periods can be pretty unpredictable, and if your migraines are triggered by hormones, you'll probably notice that they change, too. Unfortunately, for 45 per cent of women, migraines will get worse with menopause.

If you get menopausal symptoms like hot flushes and mood swings, your doctor might give you hormone replacement therapy (HRT) to help. The role that HRT plays is to add some hormones back into your body to help ease you into menopause and allow you time to adjust to it. Then you can slowly reduce the amount of HRT you're taking without suffering with the same symptoms. There are different types of HRT, such as patches and creams, which usually contain oestrogen and another hormone called progestogen. While headaches can be a side-effect of HRT, the constant dose of oestrogen might also help with your migraines.

'It's certainly worth trying HRT if you have no counter-indications,' says Professor Grossman. 'You can go on HRT and taper it off to let your body adjust naturally over months.'

So if you've found menopause to be a bit of a shock to the system and your migraines have become worse, speak to your GP about whether HRT might help. Dr Ahmed suggests that HRT with low-strength oestrogen can be better for women who live with migraines and have gone through menopause, as high-strength oestrogen HRT had been known to trigger attacks.

That said, there is some light at the end of the menopausal tunnel. Technically, you've gone through the menopause when you haven't had a period for 12 months, although it can take up to another five years for your hormones to completely settle down. But once you've gone through menopause, there's a good chance that you'll get fewer – if any – migraines.

'A lot of women do get better after menopause,' says Dr Ahmed. So if perimenopause has caused your migraines to go haywire, it's pretty reassuring to know that once your hormones settle, your migraines very well could too.

How Can You Balance Your Hormones at Home?

After reading all that, it probably seems like hormonal migraines are as unavoidable as your period itself. After all, because your hormones are inside your body, you're stuck with them. It's true that hormones aren't something that you can avoid as easily as some other triggers, such as processed meats or bright sunlight. But don't worry, that doesn't mean you're doomed to suffer because of your hormones. Yes, when it comes to triggers, hormones are a big one, but remember, often migraines are a reaction to more than one trigger at a time. So instead of seeing yourself as destined to have to cope with migraines month in and month out, try turning this situation on its head. You've now got a powerful weapon against your migraines because you know when some of them are going to strike. This is especially useful for women who have regular cycles.

- **Keep a Diary**

  Yes, this again. If it's being repeated, then it must be important, so pay attention! Keeping track of both your periods and your migraines in a diary for at least three months will help you to figure out what days your hormones are likely to be playing havoc with your head. Then you can use that diary to schedule in some migraine-avoidance time. This is when you should be kind to yourself and make sure that you avoid other triggers for a few days.

  Let's say you know that you're likely to get your period around Sunday the 15th this month, and you've also worked out that alcohol, oversleeping and the smell of coffee can trigger your migraines. Now, unless you're tackling it with help from your GP, that annoying oestrogen dip before your period is going to happen whether you like it or not. That's the bit that you can't change, so you've got to work around it. For example, those plans that you've made to go out for drinks on the Friday night with friends, followed by a lie-in and strong coffee on the Saturday morning? You can choose to rearrange them. By not exposing yourself to other triggers, you're softening the blow of the oestrogen dip trigger.

  Keeping track of your periods means that you can also be prepared with anything you'll need in case you do get an attack and react quickly with anything that helps, from medication to drinking water and getting plenty of rest. If you've kept your diary clear, it also means that you won't have the disappointment of having to cancel plans that you were looking forward to.

- **Eat the Right Things**

  Eating well is always important for migraine prevention, but particularly when you think your hormones are triggering attacks. Nutritionist Claudine Mules says that if you want to keep your hormones in check, then you should eat foods that can help to keep your blood sugar levels balanced. 'This will in turn reduce insulin, cortisol and adrenaline levels and allow other sex hormones to be made instead,' says Claudine.

  Even if your hormones aren't a concern, keeping your blood sugar balanced is good for migraine prevention in general, so this is a win-win approach. You'll read more about the effect that your diet can have on your migraines in the next chapter, but as a little preview, if you want to maintain balanced blood sugar it's a good idea to avoid sugar, processed foods and caffeine as much as possible. Instead you should opt for small portions of carbohydrates like brown rice, as well as protein such as chicken or nuts, with each meal. Also include lots of healthy fats like olive oil in your diet.

  'And 1-2 tablespoons of ground flaxseeds a day can really help balance excess oestrogen and testosterone,' says Claudine. If you haven't tried ground flaxseeds before, it's really easy to add them to smoothies, cereal, salads and stews to get that amount into your daily diet.

- **Sleep Well**

  We already know that sleep is important for keeping migraines at bay, but chances are your hormones are doing a good job of trying to keep you awake. A study done by the National Sleep Foundation in the US found that 33 per cent of women have sleep problems during the week of their period, 84 per cent of pregnant women struggle with insomnia and 20 per cent of perimenopausal women have disrupted sleep thanks to hot flashes. So, if you're going through a time like this, it's worth trying out the sleep hygiene tips we've already talked about to try to get the best rest that you can.

- **Exercise**

  'Exercise can help make periods lighter and less painful,' says Professor Grossman. 'We're not really sure of the reason why, but PMT can be evened out.'

  In fact, researchers at Khorasgan Azad University found that 30 minutes of exercise done three times a week for eight weeks reduces PMT.

So even though experts haven't worked out the finer details of why this happens, if your migraines are hormone-related, some gentle exercise just might help. But remember to be patient and allow some time for it to take effect.

My Migraines
Amy, 34

> *'I started getting migraines when I first went on the Pill. They made me feel weak and shaky, with a headache that felt like my brain was ripping apart. Within the next two years, I'd switched to the mini pill and was having several migraines each week, which meant that I found it difficult to hold down a job. They were so bad, I couldn't even roll over without being sick.*
>
> *'I don't take any hormonal contraception anymore, and I know I get migraines when my oestrogen levels are low so I've been tracking my cycles with a diary. Although I still get migraines once or twice a month, I can manage them a lot better than I used to. I know now that I crave chocolate and junk food beforehand and sometimes I get really hot and sweaty the day before a migraine. Then I get a slight headache with a very stiff neck as a warning symptom. If I feel that starting, I take some ibuprofen. Sometimes that can prevent a migraine, but if I manage to keep them at bay for two or three months, eventually they'll come back with a vengeance and I'll get a really bad one.'*

Chapter Six

FOOD AND DRINK

'It was only once I had some medication that helped with my migraines that I'd realised dehydration and not eating regularly were triggers for me.'

Jason, 46

Eat Well

Like sleep, when it comes to diet and migraines, the first thing you need to do is get the basics right. And for you, just like for anyone else, that simply means eating well. After all, you need to fuel your body with the right stuff in order to get it functioning at its best.

It's all pretty standard stuff and, in general, your diet shouldn't be much different from someone who doesn't live with migraines. You still need complex carbohydrates like brown rice and wholemeal bread, lots of protein that you'll find in foods like red meat, eggs and nuts, and plenty of fruit and veg.

On top of that, you should make sure that you get healthy fats in your diet as well, such as essential fatty acids. Your body can't make essential fatty acids itself, but they're important for heart health, cancer prevention and healthy joints. You'll find these essential fatty acids in oily fish, nuts and seeds. Other healthy fats are in foods like avocado, olive oil and unrefined, unheated seed and nut oils. And, of course, it's important to limit the amount of saturated fat and sugar that you eat in foods like crisps and cakes.

Have a look at the chart later on in this chapter for a better idea on the sorts of foods that make up a healthy diet and how much of each you should eat in a day.

Drinks Matter, Too

While we're talking about your diet, we can't ignore what you drink. And it's quite simple, really. If you want to avoid migraines, you have to drink enough to stay hydrated. It's no secret that dehydration can cause headaches and for someone who's prone to migraines, it can trigger one, too. We're not only talking about extreme dehydration here, but also the slight dehydration that it's easy to tip into on a busy day. Most of us forget to drink and get a little dehydrated from time to time. But remember that because of your migraines you're more sensitive than most people and drinking just a little bit more water can sometimes make the difference between a good day, and a migraine day.

So, what do you need to do? Just drink regularly throughout the day. Registered Nutritional Therapist Claudine Mules says that you should drink at least six glasses – or two litres – a day. Water's best, but herbal teas and vegetable juices count, too. But steer clear from caffeinated drinks like coffee and tea, which are dehydrating. 'A good tip is to drink enough so your urine is clear,' says Claudine. Easy.

And if you do feel any symptoms of mild dehydration – like feeling really thirsty, having a dry mouth, a mild headache or not needing the loo very often – have another drink. It might sound obvious but it's easy to forget that when you're exercising or ill, when the weather's hot, or when you've been drinking alcohol, you need more fluids in order to say hydrated. This is even more important if you know that dehydration can be a trigger for you.

Keep Your Blood Sugar Balanced

Have you ever left it too long between meals, and felt a real low? That horrible, grumpy, hungry, tired and even shaky feeling that disappears as soon as you munch on an apple? That's your blood sugar levels dipping. And you won't be surprised to hear that it can trigger a migraine.

Blood sugar is the amount of glucose in your blood. When you eat carbohydrates, your body converts this food into glucose, which is carried around in your blood and gives you energy. And keeping your blood sugar levels relatively stable is important for keeping migraines at bay. Fortunately, that's not a hard thing to do.

'In order to keep blood sugar levels stable, it is important to ensure that protein is eaten with each meal, ideally before the carbohydrate component,' says Claudine. 'Including healthy fats can also help slow down the conversion of food into blood sugar.'

You might have heard of high- and low-GI foods. GI stands for glycaemic index, which is a score given to different foods depending on how quickly and how much they raise your blood sugar. You digest high-GI foods really quickly and they make your blood sugar soar before crashing back down again, which isn't going to help you stay balanced. Low-GI foods, on the other hand, are digested slowly and allow your blood sugar to rise at a steadier rate. It's these low-GI foods that you need to include in your diet in order to stay on an even keel.

Foods such as biscuits and white bread have a high-GI and will be digested super-quickly, giving you that sugar high. You're better off choosing nutrient-rich low-GI foods like oats, brown rice and wholemeal pasta, which take a bit more time to move through your digestive system. Claudine also recommends including cinnamon and foods that contain chromium, such as potatoes in their skins, beef, fresh veg and cheese, in your diet to help keep your blood sugar levels balanced.

Now, when it comes to blood sugar, it's not just what you eat, but also when and how much you eat that's important. After all, skipping meals can be a migraine trigger and that's because when you haven't eaten for hours and hours your blood sugar levels plummet, leaving you vulnerable to an attack. Exactly how long it takes for this to happen can be different for everyone.

Just like eating too little, stuffing yourself silly isn't a good idea, either. That's because gorging on a massive gut-busting meal can make your blood sugar spike – even if you're eating all the right foods. And that means you risk triggering a migraine, too.

So, what can you do? Keep your food intake balanced throughout the day. Eating three proper meals a day with two or three low-carb or high-protein snacks in-between, such as a handful of nuts or some hummus and crudités, will keep things ticking away nicely without making your blood sugar levels bounce up and down like a rubber ball. Keeping track of your portion sizes is another good way to make sure that you're getting what you need.

And that leads us nicely into this handy chart, which tells you what you should be eating throughout the day, and how much, in order to have a healthy diet:

Food Type	Portion Size	How Often
Dairy or dairy substitutes Milk, cheese, yogurt (or dairy free options), as well as sesame seeds, tofu, figs and sardines with bones	Cheese – the size of both thumbs side-by-side Milk – one 200ml glass Yogurt – a small pot	Three times a day

Fruit As many different colours of fruit as possible throughout the day to get the most nutrients	You should be able to fit one portion of fruit inside your hand when it's cupped like a scoop, or half of that amount if it's dried fruit	Two to three portions a day
Vegetables Like fruit, eat a rainbow of vegetables every day	A portion of vegetables would also fit into the palm of your cupped hand	Ten portions a day
Protein Fish, red meat, poultry, tofu, nuts, eggs, seeds	The size of your palm when your hand is flat	One portion with each meal
Carbohydrates Brown rice, pasta, bread	No more than twice the size of your palm	One portion with each meal
Drinks Water, herbal tea, vegetable juice	At least 6 glasses/2l a day	Drink regularly throughout the day. You know you're having enough if your urine is clear

My Migraines
Jason, 46

'I remember having bad headaches when I was 10, or even younger. At the time, it was thought that they were sinus headaches, but looking back now I wonder if I had migraines even then. I was in my late 20s by the time I first spoke to doctors about migraines. When I had a migraine, it would feel like my entire head was an ache from the inside. I often felt sick and foggy-headed, and I didn't like bright lights, either.

'My migraines stopped when I was in my mid-30s and I was given blood pressure medication. The doctor said the medication could have this effect, and fortunately it did. However, it was only then that I looked back at what I'd been through and I realised that dehydration and not eating regularly were triggers for me.'

Are Some Foods a Trigger?

According to the Migraine Trust, around ten per cent of people who live with migraines find that food can trigger attacks. And if you're in this ten per cent and you know which foods trigger your migraines, you're pretty lucky. No, really. After all, you have the option to control what food goes in your mouth, which means that you can simply avoid your trigger outright. People whose attacks are triggered by changes in the weather or strong smells would probably trade with you in a heartbeat. Of course, if processed meats are a trigger for you, it's not fair that you can't enjoy your favourite sausage casserole without winding up in bed for two days. But before you indulge, stop and think. Are a few moments of savouring a tasty casserole really worth two days of agony and vomiting? Probably not.

After reading that, you might be crossing your fingers and hoping that you can discover a food trigger because it'll make things so much easier. If you Google it, you'll find loads of foods listed as triggers, and some of them have been mentioned later on in this chapter, too. But it's a bit of a controversial subject because there's no definitive list of food triggers.

'Most of the learned food triggers are from people describing them,' says Dr Ahmed. 'However, there are evidences of some food items that are linked with migraines.'

What that means is that not all possible food triggers have been proven in scientific studies. But just because something hasn't been found by researchers to be a trigger doesn't mean that it can't be. If you've found that you get migraines after eating chocolate and cheese and, when you give them up, your migraines stop, then it sounds as if it's likely they do trigger your attacks. And by all means, stick with what you're doing. However, be aware that there's a chance it could be a coincidence, or there may even be a warning symptom that appears to be a trigger. And it's best to fully understand which one you're dealing with.

Trigger or Warning Symptom?

Of course, if you've noticed that you get a migraine after eating certain foods, those foods might be a trigger. But they might also be your warning symptoms playing tricks on you and giving you cravings which make you eat that food in the first place. If that's the case, it's not actually a trigger at all because by the time you're eating that food, your migraine's already started. You just don't know it yet.

For example, let's say there's a lady called Donna who gets migraines. One afternoon, Donna's really craving some chocolate. She eats the chocolate and doesn't think about it again until a few hours later when a migraine starts. The same thing happens a couple of weeks on and again a few weeks after that. Before long, Donna's convinced that the chocolate has been triggering her migraines.

The trouble is, Donna's missing the big picture. When she was trying to figure out what triggered her migraine, she thought back as far as the chocolate she ate, but not the reason why she ate it. It's the craving for sweets and chocolate that are important here, rather than the chocolate itself.

What's more, it's not a trigger, either, it's a symptom – a warning symptom. The fact that Donna had eaten the chocolate is neither here nor there because her migraine was already on its way. This isn't just the case for chocolate, either, because craving savoury foods can be a warning symptom, too. So your symptoms could be sending you messages that are easy to misinterpret.

That's not to say there aren't exceptions. After all, there are hundreds of possible migraine triggers, who's to say that yours aren't triggered by chocolate? But if you think they are, it might be worth taking a closer look, just in case. It may just be a warning symptom and if you look back even further at what you were doing before the craving started, you might find that you have other triggers that you hadn't spotted before.

So How Do You Find Out if Food is a Trigger for You?

Working out any triggers – especially food triggers – can be a tricky job that requires some real detective work. So, use your migraine diary and keep note of what you've eaten before a migraine hits. If a certain food is a trigger for you, the migraine could happen within hours, or it could take as long as a couple of days. And you'll get a migraine every time you eat it, too. Often, you'll know instinctively that a certain food is a problem for you and you may already be avoiding it for that reason.

When it comes to food triggers, remember to think of the whole picture and look at what else was going on at the time. Just reviewing your diet without, for example, thinking about whether you were overtired or skipping your usual exercise routine at the time, could make you think that the ham sandwich you'd gobbled up at lunchtime was to blame when actually there were other triggers at work all along.

If after doing all that, it still looks like, say, processed meats are triggering your migraines, the next step is, of course, to stop eating all processed meats for a while. 'Ideally remove suspected triggers from the diet for two weeks,' advises Claudine. 'Then reintroduce one food at a time for a period of three days for each food.'

If, over this time, you get fewer migraines, or none at all – bingo – you've worked out a trigger. However, your work isn't done yet. Remember to keep up with your migraine diary because if you find there's no change or that your migraines creep back in, you can then use your diary to look out for other triggers. It may just be that something altogether different was the culprit all along.

Don't forget that while you're doing all this you also need to make sure you still eat a balanced diet every day. So, for example, replace the protein in processed meats with fresh meat, eggs or nuts. And pay particular attention if you're eliminating dairy foods. In this case, Claudine advises that you make sure to get your daily calcium intake from other sources, like calcium-fortified dairy-free milks, yogurts and cheeses, sesame seeds, tahini, figs, tofu and sardines with bones.

Alcohol

Anyone – even people who don't live with migraines – can get a headache after drinking alcohol. But as you're prone to headaches anyway, you might be more sensitive to alcohol, too. Whether certain alcoholic drinks are more likely to cause migraines than others seems to be a very individual thing. Some people say that they get migraines after drinking red wine or beer, while others have found it's white wine that triggers attacks.

Cured Meats

There's something known as a hot dog headache, which is, not surprisingly, a headache you get after eating a hot dog or other cured, or processed, meats, like bacon or packaged sliced turkey. It's because of the chemical compounds which are used as preservatives in the meat called nitrates and nitrites. You can find these preservatives in salted fish and pickles, too.

These chemicals are often harmless and when you eat them they just get excreted from the body without causing any problems. That is, unless you've got a shortage of Vitamin C or you don't have enough antioxidants in your body. Then these preservatives get converted into a compound called nitrosamine and it's this compound which can be more harmful to you.

It all sounds pretty complicated, but actually, there's a really easy solution. 'As vegetables contain fibre, antioxidants, vitamins, and minerals,' says Claudine, 'eat some salad with your sausage roll!' This will help to neutralise the preservatives in the cured meat. If that doesn't work for you, try avoiding processed meats altogether for two weeks to see if it helps.

Caffeine

Remember when we talked about the things that could be both triggers and treatment? Caffeine is a big one, and it's definitely something that you should keep in mind when you're working out how to prevent your migraines. But did you know that you could turn to caffeine if you feel an attack starting to come on, too? This isn't just the caffeine in your coffee or tea, but also in any chocolate you eat, certain painkillers you might be taking, and a plant called guarana, which you might find in some soft drinks.

Let's talk about prevention first. Caffeine is something that we tend to reach for out of habit, whether it's first thing in the morning, as a break during the day or as a pick-me-up when we need a boost. And it's really easy for the amount of caffeine you're having to add up throughout the day without you even realising that it's happening. But having a lot of caffeine in your diet isn't great for someone who gets migraines. Why? Because of that all-important balance that you're trying to find. Caffeine is a drug, it's a stimulant. Yes, it makes you feel more alert and awake when you first have it, but as the next hours pass, the caffeine will leave your system and those feelings will start to dip. And, of course, when it comes to migraine prevention, highs and lows are more likely to trigger attacks than a smooth, steady ride.

Caffeine withdrawal is a thing, too, and it's not just for hard-core espresso drinkers. If you have caffeine regularly – your morning coffee, for example – and you skip a day, or even just have your coffee a bit later in the morning than usual, you could risk triggering a migraine. Now, that won't be the case for everyone, and it doesn't necessarily mean you that can never have a cup of coffee again. Being aware of how caffeine affects you and your migraines is the key to working out how much you can tolerate each day.

The general advice for caffeine consumption for the average healthy person is that 400mg of caffeine a day, or the amount in about four cups of coffee, is OK. But in reality, not everybody can handle that much. 'Obviously if caffeine is a trigger it should be avoided,' says Claudine. 'Maintaining stable blood sugar levels is so important for migraine sufferers and caffeine increases cortisol and adrenaline levels, which will have a knock-on effect on blood sugar levels, so really abstaining would be best. At the very least have your caffeine *after* food to minimise the impact.'

The fact is that some people can tolerate caffeine better than others. That said, if you're spending half of your wages on coffee or finding that your recycling bin is clattering with empty energy drink cans at the end of the week, you probably already know that you could cut back. Although it's better to cut down gradually than to go cold turkey as that can also trigger a migraine. Claudine recommends cutting down by one cup a day, then switching to green tea before going completely caffeine-free. If you do get a caffeine withdrawal headache as you're tapering it off, it should settle within a couple of days.

If the idea of leaving coffee or tea behind completely is too much to bear, another option would be to try switching to decaf. While this might work for you, keep in mind that your decaf tea and coffee will still have up to 20mg of caffeine in each cup. If you want to completely eliminate caffeine from your diet, you could give herbal teas or roobios tea a try.

At this point, you might feel like caffeine is an enemy that you need to avoid at all costs. However, when it's used at the right time, it can actually be your best ally against a migraine. Experts don't know everything about how caffeine affects the brain, but they do know that caffeine causes the blood vessels in the brain to constrict, that it is a mild painkiller, and that it also boosts the effectiveness of your pain relief tablets. Which is why some people who live with migraines reach for a strong cup of coffee or a Coke during the warning or aura phases of their migraines. You may also find that you crave caffeinated drinks as a migraine's settling in. And that a shot of caffeine at the right time could actually ease your migraine, or even put a stop to it altogether.

What About Food Allergies?

The term 'food allergy' is thrown around a lot, and often used incorrectly. Technically, a food allergy is a very specific type of immune system reaction to certain foods. It can often come on within minutes of eating what you're allergic to, and can give you a rash, make your mouth tingly and itchy, cause swelling in your mouth or throat, and make you wheezy or sick. In very severe cases food allergies can be life-threatening.

Often when people talk about food allergies, they really mean food intolerances or sensitivities, like lactose or gluten intolerance. These intolerances can sometimes take hours to cause a reaction, and they can make you feel bloated, give you stomach pain, rashes and diarrhoea. And yes, headaches, too.

In one UK study done by the University of York and YorkTest, 5,000 people who suffered from food intolerance eliminated the foods from their diets that had been causing the problems for three months. And 78 per cent of them found their migraine symptoms improved.

Your migraine diary can also show if you might have developed a food intolerance or sensitivity. Look for patterns in what you've eaten and any

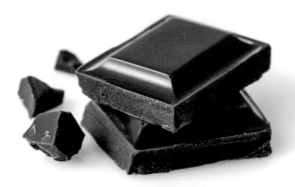

Some people believe that chocolate triggers their migraines, but craving chocolate might actually be an early warning symptom.

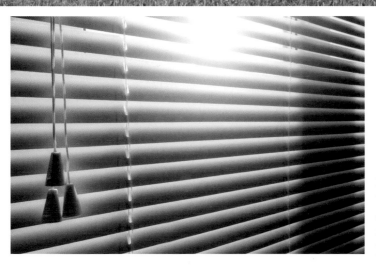

Migraines and photophobia – an aversion to light – go hand in hand around 80 per cent of the time.

Experts don't know why but looking at stripes can trigger migraines in some people.

Sensitive to light? Keep a pair of shades in your migraine survival kit.

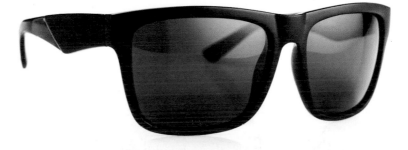

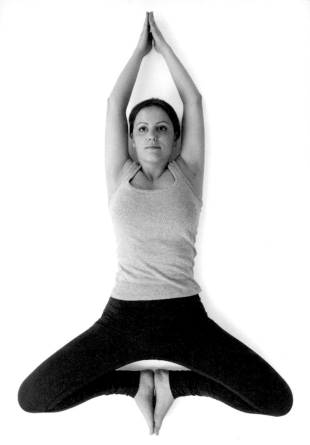

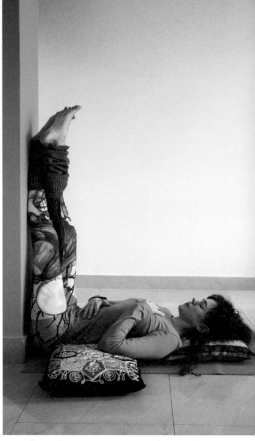

Yoga for Migraines: Supta Baddha Konasana

Yoga for Migraines: Legs up the Wall

Yoga for Migraines:
Child's Pose

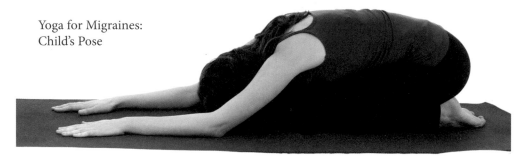

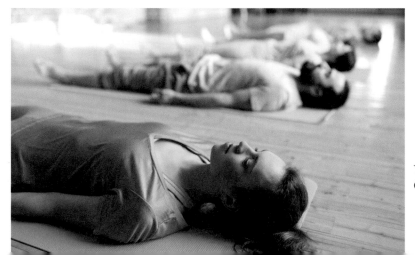

Yoga for Migraines:
Corpse Pose

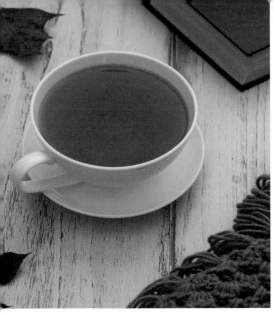

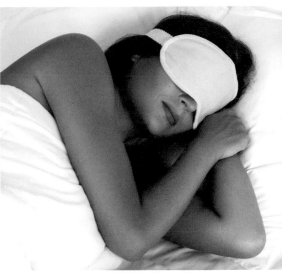

Research shows that tea drinkers can calm down more quickly after a period of stress. That's good to know if stress is a trigger for you.

Eye masks can block out light when you're feeling sensitive during an attack.

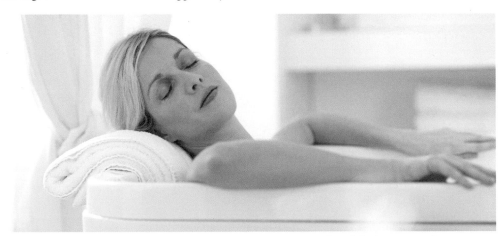

Good sleep hygiene can help to prevent migraines. For a good night's sleep, try taking a warm bath before bed.

The Pill can also help, as it can balance out your horomones.

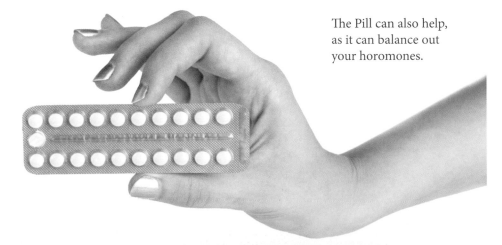

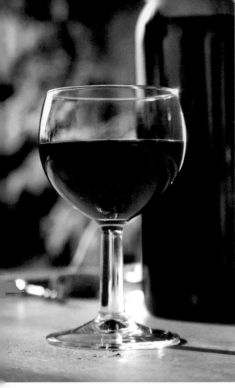

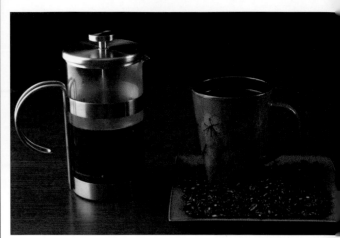

Grabbing a strong cup of coffee when a migraine hits might ease the pain.

Alcohol is a common migraine trigger.

A hot dog headache comes on after eating cured meats.

Although eating some veg with your hot dog can help.

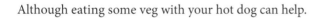

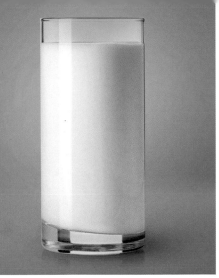

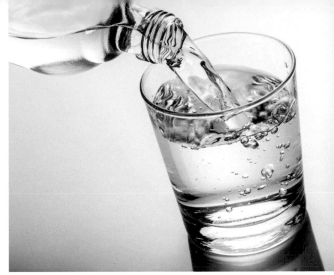

A good diet is important for preventing migraines. Make sure to include healthy foods like three portions of dairy a day.

Dehydration can be a trigger so drink at least two litres of water a day.

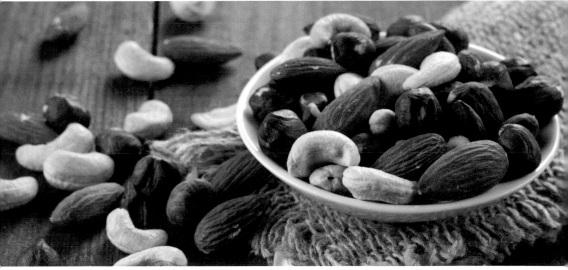

If you're avoiding processed meats, try adding nuts into your diet. They're packed with protein.

Sometimes exercise can trigger migraines but don't hang up your trainers for good.

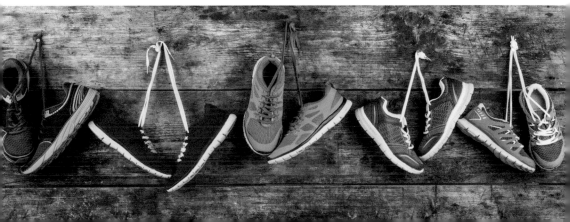

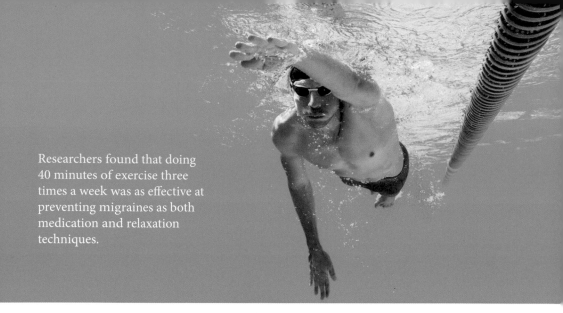

Researchers found that doing 40 minutes of exercise three times a week was as effective at preventing migraines as both medication and relaxation techniques.

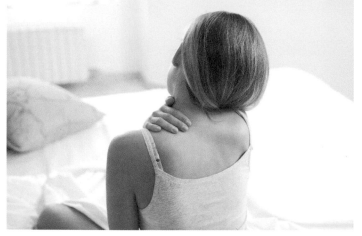

Some experts believe that neck pain is a migraine symptom rather than a trigger.

Be sure to stretch it out to avoid muscle pain after exercise.

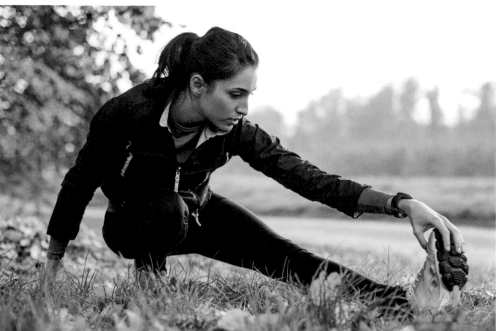

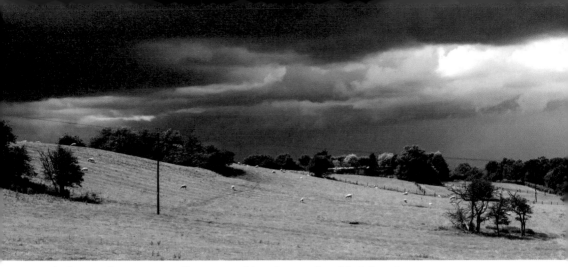

Watch the weather, storms rolling in could make your head feel thundery, too.

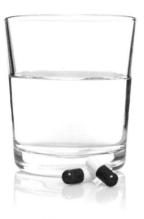

Finding the right migraine medication for you can be a matter of trial and error.

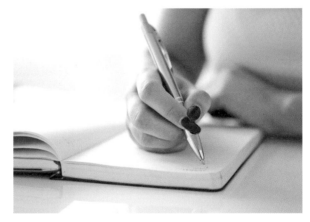

Your migraine diary is your best tool for tracking triggers.

If you're sensitive to sound, try adding soft furnishings to echoey rooms.

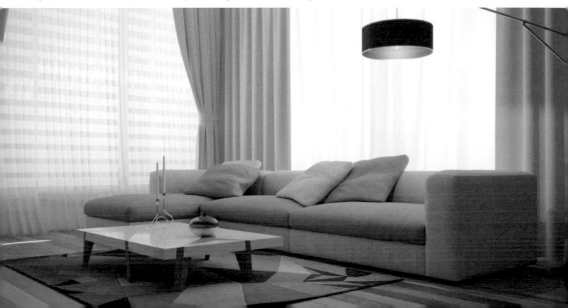

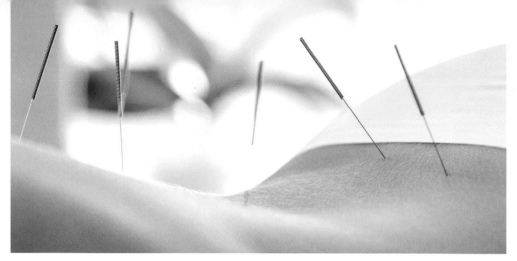

Acupuncture might help reduce your attacks and make them less severe.

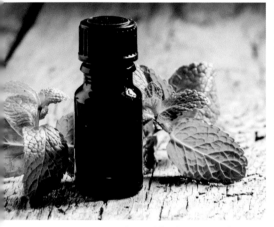

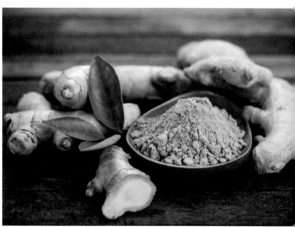

Peppermint oil can block out unpleasant smells when your nose is feeling sensitive.

Ginger powder can relieve migraines and keep nausea at bay.

You might crave caffeine, like in a glass of Coke, at the start of a migraine.

Some people find that the smell of strong perfume can be a migraine trigger.

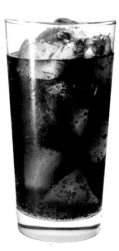

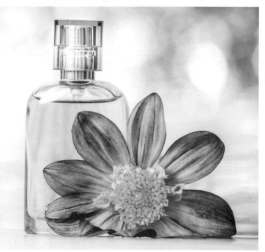

symptoms that you might have. If you suspect an intolerance, try eliminating the food or foods that might be troubling you for two weeks, then reintroduce them one at a time as Claudine advised when we talked about food triggers. And remember that you still need to make sure that you don't miss out on important nutrients in the meantime.

Word of Mouth – Food and Drink Triggers

These foods and drinks are often talked about as possible migraine triggers:

Caffeine

Chocolate

Monosodium Glutamate (MSG)

Nitrates, in foods like cured meats

Cheese, particularly aged cheese like Camembert or Blue Cheese

Alcohol, especially red wine and beer

Aspartame, a sweetener found in things like diet drinks and chewing gum

Soft drinks like squash

Any foods you may have a sensitivity to, such as dairy or gluten

Citrus fruits

My Migraines
Katherine, 35

'I've had migraines for as long as I can remember. When I have one, it feels like my skull is being squeezed. Painkillers don't help and I don't like the side-effects of prescription drugs so I've always just had to ride them out. Thankfully I don't get them as often as I did when I was a child, although they were less severe when I was young.

'I've learned that my migraines are triggered by a few things, like hormones, or if I travel somewhere with high altitude. When I was 10 my mum took me to both the GP and a homeopathist for help. The homeopathist suggested cutting out foods that have anything to do with cows, such as milk and beef, but that didn't prevent my migraines. Then my mum took the lead and tried cutting out different things from my diet for two weeks at the time. Weirdly, we found that if I didn't drink

orange squash I got fewer attacks. I have no idea what ingredient it is in the squash that triggers my migraines but avoiding it has really helped. I've had the odd glass of squash in the past 25 years and I've always regretted it!'

Can Some Foods Prevent Migraines?

That's a good question, and experts are working towards finding an answer. There has been study after study looking into the effects of certain nutrients on migraines and whether people who live with migraines have certain common vitamin or mineral deficiencies. There are no definitive guidelines yet, but researchers are continuing to work on it.

One study which shows some of the progress that has been made in this area was done at the Cincinnati Children's Hospital Medical Center. Researchers looked at vitamin deficiencies in children, teenagers and young adults with migraines and they found that many of them had mild vitamin D, riboflavin and coenzyme Q10 deficiencies. There have also been several studies done on the effects of magnesium on the prevention and treatment of migraines. In one of these, German researchers found that taking 600mg of magnesium for 12 weeks reduced the number of attacks the participants had by 41.6 per cent. Before you reach for masses of magnesium tablets, you should be aware that it's a pretty high dose, and it can cause diarrhoea and stomach trouble.

Does all this mean that everyone with migraines needs to top up on these nutrients? It's not clear yet and experts need to do more research to find out for sure.

So what does that mean for you in the meantime? Well, first of all, there's no magic menu that will make your migraines disappear. When it comes to diet and migraines, the best clear advice at the moment is that you should eat well and eat regularly.

Still, your mind might be wandering back to that research mentioned above. It's hard to ignore the idea that getting certain nutrients into your body might just help. So let's talk about those nutrients in a bit more detail to give you have a better understanding of the ones that experts are honing in on for their research, and how you can get more of them if you choose to.

Are Supplements the Answer?

When you hear that people who live with migraines might be lacking in certain nutrients, you might be tempted to rush out to your local health food store and stock up on supplements on the off-chance that they may be able to help. After all, the need to get some relief from your migraines can be a pretty powerful feeling. And wouldn't it be wonderful if there were a magic pill that could make it all stop? But you have to tread carefully here. Supplements can have side-effects and they can interfere with other medications that you're taking, so not everyone can start taking them on a whim. Also, you have to be careful if you have another condition, such as blood disorders, diabetes or if you're pregnant. So, if you do choose to try taking some supplements in addition to eating well to see if they can help to give you some migraine relief, you may want to have a word with your doctor before starting them, just in case.

Now, while we're thinking about buying some supplements, let's not forget that what we're trying to do here is keep migraines at bay without shelling out loads of money. So you're not going to find advice on the latest trends in expensive pills and potions to supplement your diet in order to help you to stay migraine-free. The point is that you shouldn't have to remortgage your house in order to feel well. But, if you want to try taking supplements, and you don't mind buying them, there are some which may be beneficial.

Calcium and magnesium are minerals that work in synergy, which means that they work together in the body. Taking a calcium and magnesium supplement – rather than one or the other on its own – will help these minerals to work as a team. Unfortunately, you may need to take supplements that have up to that high dose of 600mg of magnesium for at least three months in order to see the benefit.

'The balance is important and taking calcium/magnesium together as a supplement can ensure this balance is more likely to be attained,' says Claudine. 'Magnesium is essential in the management of the excitatory and inhibitory neurotransmitters in the brain and can bring relief and prevent occurrence of migraines when taken in therapeutic amounts that would be hard to take in via diet alone.'

Claudine also recommends a decent B-complex vitamin because B vitamins do so many things that can be beneficial for those of us who live with migraines, such as helping to control your body's stress reaction, keeping your nerves healthy and creating the feel-good chemical serotonin in your brain.

If you do decide to take supplements, the time of day that you take them and what you eat with them are very important in order to make sure that they get properly absorbed into your body. Of course, read the label of anything that you buy to see whether or not it should be taken with food. Claudine also says that it's best to avoid taking supplements within half an hour of tea or coffee, and to take any minerals in the evening.

Migraine-Friendly Foods

While it's unfortunate that no one food is going to pull the brakes on your migraines, there are foods that are migraine-friendly, because they contain those nutrients that the experts think might just help. They also have the added bonus of generally being good for you. The chart below is a list of migraine-friendly nutrients and the foods that you can eat to get these nutrients into your body.

Nutrient	What's it for?	Eat This
Magnesium	A mineral in your body that's important for things like your blood pressure, nerve function and bones. Experts have been looking into the link between magnesium and migraines for decades, but they haven't quite figured it out yet. It may be that people with migraines have low magnesium levels – or even a magnesium deficiency – and that getting extra magnesium into your body or even treating migraines with intravenous magnesium can help.	Tofu Almonds Cashew nuts Brazil nuts Peanuts Pecans Seeds Legumes Wholegrains, especially brown rice Green leafy vegetables
Riboflavin (Vitamin B2)	Riboflavin, also known as Vitamin B2, helps produce energy for your body. One American study found that taking 400mg of riboflavin a day may be able to help reduce migraine attacks. Fifty-nine per cent of the people in the study who took riboflavin over a three month period had at least a 50 per cent reduction in attacks.	Eggs Almonds Goats cheese and yoghurt Wheatgerm Yeast extract Watercress Asparagus Cabbage Broccoli Milk Mackerel

Coenzyme Q10	Coenzyme Q10 is a substance in your body that is similar to a vitamin. It has several jobs, such as producing energy and working as an antioxidant, which means that it prevents cell damage in your body. Two small studies, done in the US and Switzerland, both showed that Coenzyme Q10 reduced the number of days that the participants were suffering with migraines over a three month period.	Oily fish such as salmon, tuna and herring Beef Poultry
Vitamin D	Vitamin D is important for healthy teeth, bones and muscles and a vitamin D deficiency may be linked to migraines. Signs of vitamin D deficiency can include bone pain and muscle weakness.	Between spring and early autumn, you should be able to get all of the vitamin D you need from sunlight. But this can be trickier as the nights draw in, and the Department of Health recommends that all adults take 10mcg of vitamin D a day in autumn and winter. You can also get vitamin D from your diet by eating - Herring Sardines Trout Mackerel Eggs

Chapter Seven

EXERCISE

'Any exercise that makes me huff and puff gives me a migraine.'

Melanie, 35

Can Exercise Trigger Migraines?

Yes, sometimes it can. But before you hang up your trainers for good, keep in mind that staying fit can help to prevent your migraines, too. As long as you choose the right kind of exercise at the right level for you.

Researchers in the Netherlands looked into it. They interviewed 103 people who suffered from migraines and found that 38 per cent of those people said their migraines had started within 48 hours of exercising. More than half of the people interviewed had stopped doing the sport that they felt was the trigger.

Let's think about that last point. If a certain type of exercise triggers your migraines, you might have decided to stop doing it. Which is fine if your migraines were being triggered by spinning classes, which you hated going to anyway. But if you love going out for bike rides, and you're worried that you might have to retire your favourite cycling shorts, there might be another answer. You may just need to approach the sport in a different way.

Usually, if your migraines start after you play sports or work out, you'll find that it's only certain kinds of very strenuous exercise that will set you off. It might be a sign that you've pushed yourself too far or gone at it too hard, and you simply need to take it a bit easier. So, before you sell your beloved squash racquet on eBay, think about whether you'd be better off taking your game down a notch instead.

Let's imagine there's a man called Steve. Steve's been letting himself get out of shape, so when a friend asks him to join his local football team, he thinks it's a good idea. Only, after working up a sweat chasing the ball around for 90 minutes – BOOM – Steve gets hit with a migraine. It seems like a coincidence until it happens again the following week.

Is football triggering Steve's migraines? Maybe. But let's look at his story a bit more closely. Steve was unfit, then he threw himself into the deep end at a football game. Chances are his migraines came on afterwards because he went at it too hard, too quickly. And that sudden, intense exercise that he wasn't used to is what triggered his attack. So it wasn't necessarily playing football itself that pushed him over his threshold, but the level that he was playing at. He might've been better off having a kickabout with some mates rather than a full-on competitive match.

You can't blame Steve, really, we've all done it at some point. You might have made a New Year's resolution to exercise, or maybe you wanted to get fit quickly for a holiday. So you suddenly took up running, or started going to boot camp. Or perhaps you pushed yourself to go for an extra-long cycle one day. And hours later, you got a migraine. This is called exercise-induced migraine and it's what happens when you do exercise that takes you past the threshold of what you can handle.

'You'd know if you had it because it would happen every time,' says Dr Ahmed. It's hardly surprising that pushing yourself too far, whether it happens in the swimming pool or on the rowing machine, can be a trigger. Migraine brains don't like abrupt change and if you've suddenly gone at it harder than usual, you're bound to be thrown off-balance. But let's not forget that balance is exactly what you need to avoid migraines. So what's the alternative? Loafing at home on the sofa because you're too frightened to work up a sweat in case it all goes wrong? You could do that, but you'd be missing out on a fantastic way to help keep your migraines at bay.

'If you don't have exercise-induced migraine,' says Dr Ahmed. 'Exercise can be helpful.' It may just be a matter of finding the right kind of exercise at the right level for you.

Ways That Exercise Helps to Prevent Migraines

In a small study done at the University of Gothenburg in Sweden, researchers found that doing 40 minutes of exercise three times a week was as effective at preventing migraines as both medication and relaxation techniques. So exercise is pretty important if you want to keep your migraines away. But how does it work?

- **Sleep**

  By now you know that staying fit helps you to sleep better, and that good sleep is important for migraine prevention. So these two things work in harmony to help keep you on an even keel. Some experts say that you shouldn't exercise in the evening as it can be too stimulating and it might actually make it more difficult for you to fall asleep at night. But do what works for you. If you find that going to the gym in the evenings after work makes you feel great, then stick with it. On the other hand, if it leaves you too wired, don't give up altogether. Change it up instead and try going early in the morning or at lunchtime to see if things improve.

- **Endorphins**

  Endorphins are pretty amazing things. They're chemicals that can be released in your body when you've worked out and as they're natural opiates, they improve your mood, relieve stress and act as natural painkillers, too. In fact, that endorphin rush after exercise feels so good that it's sometimes called a runner's high.

  If you make a habit of exercising, your body will be flooded with these feel-good painkillers on a regular basis. There was a study done by Australian researchers where they compared the pain tolerance of people who had not been exercising at all to that of people who'd been doing regular exercise for six weeks. The group who'd been exercising had increased their tolerance for pain, meaning that they could handle it better. This could be thanks to lots of changes that happen as the body gets fitter, including that all-important endorphin rush. And when it comes to migraines, that can only be a good thing.

  The gym and the swimming pool aren't the only places where you can get this natural high. You can get it in the bedroom, too. Believe it or not, researchers at the University of Munster in Germany did a study about sex and migraines. And 60 per cent of the people involved who'd had sex during a migraine said their symptoms had improved afterwards. Experts believe this could be thanks to the release of endorphins that happens during sex. Of course, having sex during a migraine isn't right for everyone. In fact, only 34 per cent of the people who were involved in the study said that they had any sexual activity during their migraines, and 33 per cent of those who did found that their attacks got worse. So it's a personal thing.

- **Healthy Weight**

  Researchers at Johns Hopkins University School of Medicine in the US compiled the results of 12 different studies on weight and migraines. They found that obese people, who are those whose BMI is higher than 30, are 27 per cent more likely to have migraines than people who are a healthy weight. Underweight people with a BMI lower than 18.5 are 13 per cent more likely to have migraines.

What does all this mean? Simply that if you're in a healthy weight range you'll be less likely to get migraines. Experts don't know yet whether gaining or losing weight will reduce the number of migraines that you get, but exercising can certainly help you to maintain your weight at a healthy level.

The Basics of Healthy Exercise

So now we know *why* you should exercise to help keep migraines away, but when you live with migraines *how* do you go about it? The same as anyone else, really. You just have to keep a closer eye on how you're feeling.

According to the Chief Medical Office, people between the ages of 19 and 64 should do two-and-a-half hours of moderate intensity exercise every week. That's the sort of exercise that gets your heart pumping, but it shouldn't be too strenuous. If it leaves you too out of breath to carry on a conversation, then you're going at it too hard. It sounds like a lot but it's really easy if you break it up into little chunks of exercise throughout your week. So, for example, your two-and-a-half hours could be made up of 30 minutes of brisk walking, cycling or swimming five days a week, or a combination of all three. Before you know it, you'll have done plenty of exercise, and you'll probably be feeling a lot better for it.

Of course, when you've got a migraine you'll be lucky if you can get out of bed. Going out for a walk, let alone a cycle or a swim, might not be an option for days on end. Your migraines could even be so frequent and disruptive that you find it difficult to motivate yourself to do any exercise at all, even on the days when you haven't had an attack. Even if you're starting from scratch, there are gentle ways to introduce a bit of exercise at times when you're feeling well enough to do it.

So how do you approach exercise when things have been tricky and you haven't done any for a long time? Start small and build it up slowly. Personal Trainer Katharine Busby, with Yes Please Fitness in Newcastle upon Tyne, says swimming, speed walking and jogging are all good options that you can consider trying if you haven't done any exercise for a while.

'The important thing with beginning exercise is to take it at a safe pace but have a progression in mind,' Katharine says. 'It's not about setting yourself some Iron Man-style challenge. It's just personal progression rather than accepting that, fitness-wise, where you are now is where you'll be forever.' In other words, take it slowly and aim to get fitter, little bit by little bit.

Katharine advises that if you want to start swimming, for example, and you find that you can do ten lengths of breaststroke now, use that as your base to build on. So, you might give yourself a goal of, say, 15 lengths of breaststroke, which you can build up to over the next month.

While you don't need to spend money on a gym membership to get fit, if you already belong to one, ask an instructor for some tips. Tell him or her about your migraines and ask for help coming up with an exercise programme that will work for you, which you can do on the days when you're feeling well enough to work out.

Whatever you've chosen to do, stick to it as best you can. Of course, this isn't easy when migraines hit and you shouldn't beat yourself up about missing out on a workout because of your disorder. Forcing yourself to go out for a walk when all you want to do is lie in bed really isn't going to help you. And, of course, there may be some attacks where you have no choice but to skip the Pilates class you'd planned to go to. That's OK. Instead, allow yourself a break to get the rest and recovery that you need, and then get back to it when you're feeling better.

'Plan when you're going to exercise at the beginning of each week,' Katharine says. 'That way, if a migraine strikes and it means you miss a session, you already know when the next one is. This will help keep you on track even if some sessions have to be missed.'

Check In With Your Body

As someone who lives with migraines, it's always a good idea to be aware of how you're feeling, whether you're on the train on your way to work or balancing upside-down at a yoga class. Sometimes, you might be just fine, and ready to take on the world. But there will also be busy days and weeks when you could slowly be getting off-kilter without even realising it.

So, before every workout, pause to have a little listen to your body. Have you noticed any warning symptoms? Are you particularly tired or run down at the moment? Have you just come through the worst of an attack, and are maybe still feeling a bit woozy or tired? If you're not feeling 100 per cent, this isn't the day to push yourself to do your longest ever cycle or lift heavy weights. Even if exercise isn't usually a trigger for you, pushing your body too far at the wrong moment is never a good idea for someone who lives with migraines. Instead, take an easy day with a gentle swim, or some relaxing yoga. Or give yourself a break and just rest for today and pick it up again tomorrow.

Even when you're doing everything right and building up your fitness gradually, you might find that some types of exercise, or exercising very intensely, can still be a trigger for you. That threshold will be different for everyone so be mindful of how you're feeling after you exercise, too. Keeping note of your exercise in your migraine diary can also help you to work out if you've pushed it too far and you need to ease off a bit. For example, you might be able to swim lengths for 20 minutes without any problems, but pushing yourself to do a 30-minute swim could trigger an attack. So next time, you can take it back to 20 minutes and enjoy your swim, migraine-free. Like anything with migraines, you need to find your balance with exercise and stay within the limits that work for you.

Migraine-Friendly Exercise

In one study, done at the University of Gothenburg in Sweden, 20 people who lived with migraines found that following a special regime on an exercise bike 3 times a week was a good way to go. During a three-month period, only one person involved had a migraine triggered by the exercise.

That said, another study, done in India, found that yoga is a good type of exercise to choose, too. This time, people who live with chronic migraines did about an hour of yoga five days a week for six weeks. The results were that they had fewer migraines, plus the attacks that they did have were less painful.

This just shows that there isn't a one size fits all workout that you can follow in order to stay balanced. Which is a good thing, actually, because it means that you can choose the type of exercise that you enjoy and that makes you feel better. Of course, if your migraines are chronic, gentle yoga would probably be much less daunting than a full-on high intensity interval training class, complete with pumping music. So unless researchers find one incredible fitness regime that helps everyone, do what works best for you. Whatever exercise you enjoy and feel good doing is the one that you should stick with.

Types of Exercise to Try

If you've decided to start a new exercise class, speak to the instructor and explain that you get migraines and you don't want to push yourself too hard. Classes like circuits are great because they can be done at a pace to suit you. You could also try -

Yoga

Pilates

Walking

Swimming

Cycling

Dance classes

Zumba

Feed Your Workouts

Remember your blood sugar levels, and how important it is to keep them steady? That goes for when you're playing sports, too. Between 30 and 90 minutes before you exercise, Katharine says that it's important to have a meal or a snack that's healthy but contains fast-release carbs that will help to keep your energy up throughout your workout. She suggests trying a banana, Greek yogurt with dried fruit or a smoothie.

Once you've finished your workout, you'll want to have a nibble within 90 minutes afterwards, too. This time, Katharine says it's good to choose slow-release carbs, like brown rice, wholemeal bread or non-starchy vegetables such as green beans or asparagus, with lean protein, such as cottage cheese, beans, or chicken. This will be great for stopping your blood sugar levels from dropping after you've exercised, too.

And while you're at it, remember to keep drinking water, as well. The National Hydration Council says that you should sip water every 20 minutes when you're exercising and make sure that you keep drinking after you've finished to avoid dehydration, too. If you tend to forget to drink, Katharine suggests trying a free app like Daily Water to remind you to keep drinking throughout the day.

Support Your Neck

For some people who live with migraines, it's thought that sore neck muscles can trigger an attack. So, whether you're doing circuit training or are at a Pilates class, you need to stay mindful of your neck and any strain that it may be under. If you know it's a trigger for you, take extra care of this area and avoid doing anything that puts strain on your neck, like sit-ups with your hands clasped behind your head.

Also, be aware that it's not just overdoing it at the gym that can cause neck pain. If you know that a pain in the neck can become more than, well, a pain in the neck, stay mindful of it at other times, too. Simple things that lots of us do every day, such as carrying a handbag weighed down with too much stuff on your shoulder or lifting a toddler out of his cot awkwardly, can cause your neck to tense up, so if neck pain can be a trigger for you, be aware and take care. Think about how you do everything, from taking your shopping into the house, to carrying your suitcase at the airport, to how you're sitting at your computer and protect your neck at all times.

That said, some experts believe that neck pain is actually a symptom of migraine, rather than a trigger. So if you find that your neck tends to ache before the attack phase hits, you may want to take your medication as soon as you feel that first niggle.

Easy Ways to Avoid Neck Pain

- **Think About Your Posture**

Good posture helps to prevent neck pain. It's as simple as that. When you're standing with good posture, your head will be straight, your shoulders will be back and your weight will be distributed evenly between both of your legs. But there are so many things in day to day life that can lead to poor posture, such as having your computer screen at the wrong height, standing for long periods of time in high heels and sleeping on your stomach. All of these things can cause your neck to ache.

- **Stretch It Out**

If you get a sore neck, Pauline Gibbons, owner of Tring Yoga Studio, advises doing very gentle, slow neck circles, shoulder shrugs and shoulder circles regularly throughout the day – as often as every hour or so. Don't wait until it hurts to start, it's better to do the exercises before you get neck pain to keep everything loose.

No Pain, No Pain

The one thing that you don't want to get out of your new exercise regime is more pain, particularly as sore muscles can be a migraine trigger for some people. So as well as building up your regime slowly, make sure that you warm up before working out and cool down afterwards to help stay pain and injury-free.

When you warm up you're slowly increasing your heart rate and getting some blood flowing to your muscles before you take your workout up a notch. Katharine advises doing a gentle version of your planned workout – so if you're heading out for a run, start by walking – for five minutes.

'If you think of a scale where one is lying on the sofa and 10 is running from an axe-toting murderer, you want to aim for about a four,' Katharine says. 'You can feel you're getting warmer but you're not unable to do more exercise when the warm-up is over.'

After these first five minutes, do some dynamic stretches. Dynamic stretches are those done with movement, and they help your body to stay warm while you're doing them before finally heading off on your run. Arm circles and lunges are both types of dynamic stretches that you can do once you're warmed up.

Once you've finished your workout, walk for another five minutes to cool down, this time slowly reducing your speed to allow your heart rate to come back to normal. Follow this up with some static stretches, where you stay still during the stretch, to keep your muscles from getting sore.

My Migraines
Melanie, 35

'Certain types of exercise triggers my migraines and I know that I have to be careful about what I do. I can go swimming and go for the occasional run as long as I don't push it too hard. If I don't do any sprinting, stick to a steady jog, and don't run any further than 5k, I know I'll be OK. I learned the hard way, though. I tried to get into the Insanity DVD, but it was horrendous! Each time I did it, I felt like my head was going to explode.

'I'm really careful when I'm working out because I feel like the older I get, the worse my migraines become. They start with a metallic taste in my mouth, which is my warning symptom. Then when the pain and sickness kick in, they can be so bad, I'll have to crawl on all fours just to get to the bathroom. I take Sumitriptan, which the doctor prescribed, when I feel a migraine coming on, but while one tablet used to do the trick, now I find I have to take more and more. Sometimes that doesn't even work and I have to go to the doctor for an injection of Voltarol for the pain.'

Chapter Eight

STRESS

'Stress is definitely a migraine trigger for me and I don't always sleep particularly well, which adds to the problem. A friend recommended the Headspace app and I found that I slept better and, if I kept up the habit, that I could better manage my stress, which helped with my migraines, too.'

Fiona, 33

What is Stress?

That probably sounds like a silly question. After all, who hasn't been stressed at some point? There's no doubt you've felt a moment of panic when something has gone wrong, or maybe you've had too much on and felt overwhelmed. Yes, when you Google the definition of stress, words like 'tension' and 'pressure' come up in the results. However, stress is more than that. And it's not always such a bad thing.

Stress is something you feel when there's a change or challenge in your life. Happy events, like getting married or being offered your dream job, are classed as stresses just as much as worrying times, like when you've had an argument or have just been given some bad news. In fact, eustress is the word for positive stress, which is the thrill you get from riding a rollercoaster or the high you feel when you fall in love.

Whether you're experiencing positive or negative stress, all this tension and excitement still has an impact on your body. You see, stress doesn't just affect your mind and your emotions, you have a powerful physiological reaction to it, too. When you feel stressed, your brain goes on red alert and this causes your body to be flooded with hormones like adrenaline, noradrenaline and the stress hormone cortisol. Your blood pressure goes through the roof, your digestive system slows right down and you can feel a heavy knot in your stomach or wind up drenched with sweat.

This reaction in your body is known as the fight or flight response and it's how we've evolved to deal with threatening situations. Fight or flight was exactly what cavemen, who were very likely to come face-to-face with predators, needed in order to survive. That sudden rush of energy to bolt away from the beast, or the bravery to confront it, was lifesaving. But fast-forward to modern day, and this heightened state of anxiety might be a bit over the top for getting you through a traffic jam or to the end of a rollercoaster ride.

Of course, another reaction that you can have to stress is a migraine. And, as migraines can be stressful in themselves, particularly if you get them a lot or if your symptoms are severe, your migraines could be making you more stressed, too. 'Certainly migraines can cause stress as well,' says Nicky Lidbetter, Chief Executive of Anxiety UK. 'It impacts on daily functioning, home and work life.'

The whole thing can become a bit of a vicious circle. Stress triggers your migraines, which causes more stress, and triggers more migraines. So you can see why it's so important to understand the stress in your life and find ways to stay relaxed whenever you can.

When you're stressed, it can affect your sleep, it can cause you to change your eating habits and it can lead you to drink more. That goes for exciting days as well as very bad ones. After all, when you've just been offered your dream job you may be so elated that you celebrate with champagne and then your mind races with excitement as you try to sleep. And as all of these things can also be migraine triggers, tackling stress can have an incredible impact on your life.

Stress and Migraines

'My migraines aren't triggered by stress,' you might be thinking. 'I always get them when I'm having a lovely time, like on the weekends, or on holiday.' Don't be fooled by the timing, if migraines strike in your down time, it can still mean that stress is a trigger for you. In fact, according to a study done by researchers at Montefiore Headache Center and Albert Einstein College of Medicine at Yeshiva University in New York, migraines are five times more likely to start in the six hours *after* a stressful situation. That means that as your stress levels are dropping – or even once you've chilled out again – you could be most vulnerable to an attack. Once again, it's that lack of balance that's the culprit. After all, if your stress levels didn't go sky-high in the first place, they wouldn't have to drop again, leaving you in that vulnerable situation.

Weekend Headaches

Weekend headaches are exactly what they sound like – headaches that you get on your days off. Although the stress that builds up during the week can certainly contribute to weekend headaches, there can be other triggers, too. For example, if you get up at 7am on Monday to Friday and have a cup of coffee at 7.30 like clockwork, lying in until 10am on Saturday and delaying that boost of caffeine until 10.30 can both be migraine triggers. If this is happening to you, it can help to find stress management techniques that work for you, but also follow the advice that you read about in the sleep chapter and get up around the same time each day, following the same routine. While relaxing with a lie in on your days off might sound like a nice idea, it's not so nice if you spend the entire weekend with a migraine.

My Migraines
Laura, 23

'I was going through a very stressful time nine months ago and that's when my migraines started. Doctors weren't sure what was wrong at first and they suggested that it could be things like an ear infection or a sinus infection. Eventually a neurologist diagnosed me with chronic migraine with vestibular symptoms.

'My symptoms are crazy, I've never known anything like them and I've had them 24 hours a day since they started. Occasionally I get pain and blurred vision, but most of the time it's just a strange sort of dizziness. I have this floating, bobbing sensation, like I'm detached from the world around me. It's like my head is a heavy bowling ball balanced on top of my neck and I haven't got much energy. I feel like I'm swaying when I'm standing still and I've even had a dropping sensation, as if I'm in a lift which has fallen a few feet. At one point I couldn't walk because my muscles were so weak and I felt so dizzy.

'At the moment I'm taking 20mg of amitriptyline and 75mg of topirimate at 7.30 every night before bed, and I'm making lots of lifestyle changes too, such as getting between eight and nine hours of sleep a night, drinking lots of water and making sure my diet is healthy. I also take vitamins every day, like B2 and magnesium, and I have B12 injections.

'To deal with stress, I do mindfulness and meditation. I often take baths to help me to relax, too.'

The Difference Between Stress and Anxiety

Sometimes, the words stress and anxiety can be used to describe the same thing, and anxiety can also feel like a reaction to stress. However, there's actually an important difference between the two, and it's all to do with what's going on around you at the time.

'Stress can be pinned down to something you've experienced,' says Nicky. 'Anxiety is disproportionate to the situation experienced.'

What that means is if you feel your heart pounding, you break out in a sweat or if you have sleepless nights over a major event in your life that's gone wrong, you're under stress. If you're feeling all of these things because of a slight mishap, or you're worried about something that might happen in the future, chances are you're suffering with anxiety.

So, for example, if you've been made redundant at work, it would make sense that you might have a few sleepless nights. But if everything's fine at work yet you're lying awake worrying about what might happen if you suddenly aren't able to carry on with your job, that could be down to anxiety. And anxiety can be associated with migraines, just like stress. A study done at the University of Toronto found that people with migraines are three times more likely to have Generalised Anxiety Disorder than people who don't.

Whether you find that stressful moments can trigger your migraines, or you suffer with anxiety, there are things that you can do to bring some calm and peace into your life. And this can also help you to get some relief from your migraines in the process.

Easy Ways to Keep Calm

Of course, stress is a part of life and there's no way to avoid it entirely. But when you're trying to stay balanced, you don't want your hormone levels constantly spiking, or your heart pounding with fear too often. So what can you do if stress triggers your migraines? Use calming techniques, which will help you to stay on an even keel day-to-day. These techniques also make it easier to cope with those crazy moments that happen to all of us. 'There are lots of things that you can do on a self-help basis,' says Nicky.

Think of your body as a piece of silk. When it's laid flat, it's perfectly smooth and serene, just like you on a good day. But it doesn't take much – maybe a puff of air – to cause a little ripple. A bigger gust of wind will cause the silk to flap about, wrinkle and scrunch up, which is like your body reacting to stress. So you have to constantly smooth out that silk in order to keep it as settled and peaceful as possible. And it's the same with techniques for dealing with stress.

If you make it a habit to do things every day that can help you to stay calm, you'll feel more relaxed in general, and better placed for dealing with anything that comes your way. These techniques aren't difficult and they can help when you're dealing with particularly stressful moments, too. Here are a few easy ideas to try:

- **Have a Cup of Tea**

  Seriously. Of course, it's always nice to have a cuppa, but tea isn't just relaxing because it's warming and comforting. Researchers at University College London found that drinking tea can actually help you to recover from a stressful situation more quickly. In the small study of 75 men, half were given tea and the other half were given a tea-like drink to sip over a six-week period. Then they gave the men some challenging tasks to do, which raised the stress hormone cortisol levels of both groups. Fifty minutes after the tasks, the tea-drinking men's cortisol levels had dropped by nearly twice as much as the group who'd been given the fake tea. Which shows that after periods of stress, tea drinkers are able to calm down more quickly. So go on, get the kettle on.

- **Laugh**

  It's common sense that having a laugh will make you feel less stressed. And while it may seem like a bit of a cliché, a good giggle actually lowers both your cortisol and adrenaline levels. Laughter's really great for people who live with migraines because while it's relaxing you, it also boosts those pain-killing endorphins as well. Win-win.

- **Have Sex**

  According to a study done at the University of Paisley, the blood pressure of people who have intercourse stays lower during stressful situations. That doesn't mean you have to jump in the sack the moment your stress levels skyrocket, but just that having an active sex life has a positive impact on the way you respond to stress. If you're not feeling frisky, a kiss and a cuddle is great, too. Hugging someone you love can help to keep your blood pressure down and kissing also keeps cortisol levels low.

- **Talk About It**

  If there's something on your mind, don't keep it bottled up inside. Instead, choosing to speak to a friend you trust or a family member you feel close to can help. Or, if you're struggling with anxiety, maybe you'd rather talk about it with someone who understands how you're feeling. There are plenty of self-help groups that you can go to where you can meet other people who are going through something similar, and where you can learn about the techniques they're using to cope with anxiety. You'll find a list of these groups on the Anxiety UK website (www.anxietyuk.org.uk).

Counselling can also give you a safe place to talk about the things that are troubling you. If you'd like to give it a go, you can self-refer by contacting a local counselling service directly, or your GP can work out what type of referral you need. 'If you're feeling quite low, it's not a bad thing to see your GP,' says Nicky. How long the NHS waiting list will be depends on where you live, but the wait isn't as long as it used to be, so please don't let this put you off getting some support if you need it.

Your Autonomic Nervous System

The autonomic nervous system in your body controls a lot of things that you're often not even aware of, like your digestion and your heartbeat. The two parts of this system that deal with stress are the sympathetic nervous system, which gets your body ready for the fight or flight response, and the parasympathetic nervous system, which calms you down. Let's say you've got a tight deadline on a big project at work and you're starting to panic that you'll never finish everything on time. That means your sympathetic nervous system has been stimulated. Using relaxation techniques can stimulate the parasympathetic nervous system and restore balance between the two, making it easier for you to get things done.

Three Routes to Relaxation: Mindfulness, Yoga and The Breath

Mindfulness-based stress reduction (MBSR) is a program which was first used in 1979 to help people to cope with the difficult times in their lives. MBSR uses techniques like mindfulness and yoga, and it's been found to help with a wide range of physical and emotional conditions, including migraines. One study done in the US showed that when people with migraines were given an eight-week course of MBSR, their attacks became less severe and less disabling.

Now, this might feel like a big leap into alternative methods, and it might be very new to you. But don't worry, you don't have to spend every weekend wearing stretchy yoga pants and doing chanting to use these practises to help you relax. The good news is that even the most basic mindfulness practise or simple breathing exercise can help you to feel less stressed. And if being less stressed is a way to prevent your migraines, isn't it worth a shot? The stretchy pants are optional.

Whether you call it mindfulness or just taking five, whether you're doing some relaxing stretches or giving yourself a chance to pause in the middle of a hectic day, what matters is that you're doing something to unwind and relax. And all of those little calm moments throughout the week can add up and become habit-forming. In a good way. Before you know it, your mini daily stress-busters will become a part of your day-to-day routine and you'll do them without a second thought. And you'll be a lot more relaxed for it, too.

The trick is finding a technique that works for you so that you'll stick with it. And that's why you'll find three different routes to relaxation to try here. They can all work to make you feel calmer and more balanced, it's just a matter of figuring out which one – or ones – you like best. You might even enjoy all three.

Route to Relaxation Number One: Breathe

Breathing can be a fantastic and simple technique to help keep you calm. Of course, you've been breathing all your life, but your breath isn't just a way of getting air into your lungs, it's also a tool that you can learn to use to reduce stress. Which means that the right kind of breathing can help you to prevent migraines, too.

When you're stressed, your breathing changes. Part of the fight or flight response is that your breathing gets shallower to help get more oxygen into your body. You'd need this extra oxygen if, for example, you had to run from a burning building. But if you're just having a bad day at work, you might be better off keeping a cool head rather than getting pumped up with all that oxygen. And by consciously breathing more slowly and deeply, you can make your body and your mind calmer, too.

What you're actually doing with this deep, controlled breathing is mimicking the sort of breathing that you naturally do when you're relaxed and using that to trick yourself into actually calming down. It's a sort of reverse psychology with your breath – if you breathe as if you're calm, then you start to feel calmer. Deep breathing's been used in this way for a long time, but only recently, scientists at Stanford University College of Medicine and the University of California may have found out why it works. Some research done on mice has shown that there are neurons in the brain which keep track of breathing and if the breath changes, these neurons cause an emotional reaction. So, if your breathing becomes shallow, you start to feel stressed. But if you take charge and choose to breathe more deeply, the rest will follow, too.

> **A Four-Step Breathing Exercise For Relaxation**
>
> As you do this, your body will respond by slowing your heart rate, reducing blood pressure and your cortisol levels can even drop, too. You don't even have to wait until you're super-stressed to give it a try.
>
> 1) Close your eyes and place your hand on your chest so you can feel each breath.
> 2) Breathe in through your nose and count: 'in, 2, 3, 4.'
> 3) Then hold for two counts.
> 4) Breathe out through your mouth and relax your body, counting: 'out, 2, 3, 4, 5, 6.'
> 5) Repeat.

Route to Relaxation Number Two: Mindfulness

Mindfulness has become a bit of a trendy buzzword. As it's become more popular you've probably heard of it, but it can seem like a bit of a mystery if you've never actually tried it before.

'Mindfulness is a word that has been translated from Eastern languages and adopted in the West to mean paying attention in a certain way and experiencing what is in your awareness without judgement,' explains Counselling Psychologist Dr Lisa Greenspan.

It's quite simple, really. Mindfulness is about taking a break, slowing things down for a little while – even just a few moments – and becoming aware of how you feel. Some people call it being present, others say it's about being not doing, but it all boils down to the same thing. When you practise mindfulness, you're taking the time to observe what you're feeling, both physically and emotionally. Then you can choose how you want to respond to those feelings, rather than simply reacting to them without a second thought.

For example, you might have a sore shoulder today and that could be making you grumpy and causing you to think things like: 'It's not fair that my shoulder hurts,' or 'Now I won't be able to go swimming this evening'. Keep in mind that emotions are powerful, but they're short-lived. You can use mindfulness techniques to pause and stop this stress from taking over. Then you'll have the option to choose whether you're going to continue to feel annoyed about your sore shoulder, or whether to accept that you're going to miss swimming tonight. You might even decide to make the best of it and go out for a meal with a friend this evening instead.

But you don't have to wait until the stressful moment when you're stuck in a traffic jam or have had a bad day at work to practise mindfulness. It's actually better if you don't. Instead, just being mindful for ten minutes a day can help you to handle the stress better when you do find yourself up against it. When you practise mindfulness regularly, you train your body and mind how to react more calmly. Then, when you do find stress building up, taking a moment to breathe – even just one breath taken in the stance mentioned in the ten-minute mindfulness practise below – will help you to find that familiar calm when you need it most.

'The body's nervous systems become overloaded with chemicals that won't allow us to relax when we're in situations we find stressful,' says Dr Greenspan. 'Practising mindfulness regularly can prepare the body to react differently when a stressful cue or trigger arises.'

If you were training for a marathon, you'd go out running every day so that your body and mind would be equipped to handle a big race, right? Well, this is a similar thing. Except, instead of a running race, you're training your body and mind to deal with the feeling of stress. The more well-trained you are, the easier it will be for you to handle it.

The thing to remember about mindfulness is that if you're otherwise healthy, it's safe, and it won't make your migraines worse. However, if you have mental health issues, you should ask your doctor before giving it a go.

You can feel the positive, relaxing effects of mindfulness from the first time you do it. And it's cumulative, which means the more you practise mindfulness, the more of an impact it will have. So even if you don't feel like it's something you'd normally do, it could be worth a try. It might even help.

10-Minute Mindfulness Practise

These are Dr Greenspan's four steps to a more mindful you. Take your time with each step and focus on each sensation, one at a time, before concentrating on your breathing at the end. You can take 10 minutes to do this each day, or, if you can't find 10 minutes to do it in one go, use something as a reminder to pause and take a mindful breath occasionally, like whenever you put on the kettle. Your 10 minutes will soon add up over the course of the day.

1) Spine
Stand or sit with your back against a wall if you can. Look straight ahead and lean forward slightly, then back a bit before settling in the centre, which is your neutral spine position.

2) Shoulders

The next step is to drop your shoulders. Imagine that you have a heavy suitcase in your left hand and drop your shoulder down as if the suitcase is pulling your arm towards the ground. Then, still holding that imaginary suitcase, do the same with a second one in your right hand. Come back up to centre with both pretend cases still weighing your hands down.

3) Jaw

Release any tension in your jaw by opening your mouth slightly and resting your tongue at the back of the roof of your mouth.

4) Breathe

There's nothing important to look at right now so allow your gaze to shift until your eyes are out of focus. And breathe. This is when you can become aware of any sensations in your body or emotions that you may be feeling at the moment.

Another way to try this is through guided mindfulness, which is where an expert talks you through your practise. If you'd prefer that to having a go on your own, try an app like Headspace. There are lots of free mindfulness videos on YouTube that you could check out, too.

Route to Relaxation Number Three: Yoga

We've already talked about yoga as a good exercise choice for people who live with migraines. One reason for that may be because yoga can leave you feeling calm and relaxed.

'Yoga means union,' says Pauline Gibbons, who owns Tring Yoga Studio in Hertfordshire. 'It's all about getting things to work in union – your mind, breath and body. Depending on the type of yoga you do, it can be very physically challenging or it can be relaxing.'

Yoga is more than just stretching and standing on your head, it's actually a very mindful and meditative type of exercise. After all, while you're standing on one foot with your arms in the air, you need to be focussing on how you feel at that moment to stop yourself from toppling over. Which means it gives you a chance to stop worrying about that backlog at work or the argument you had with your wife earlier in the morning. So while you're practising your tree pose, you're also taking a break from the day's stresses. You might find that you enjoy it, too.

'A lot of people think meditation is stopping all thoughts, but your mind *will* think, so it's actually just cutting down the chatter and clutter,' says Pauline. 'Yoga helps you focus on one thing and clear out your mind.'

If you belong to a gym, you can check out the yoga classes on offer there, but you don't need to leave home – or shell out for a gym membership – to give it a go. There are lots of yoga channels on YouTube, such as Yoga With Adriene, with tons of different types of free yoga videos to choose from. So even if you've never done it before, you can give a beginner's lesson a try. Make sure you ask your doctor first if you've got a medical condition or you're not sure if you're fit enough to start, though.

Simple, Relaxing Yoga Poses

Pauline advises holding each of these poses for a minimum of five minutes for a really relaxing routine:

Supta Baddha Konasana
Lie on your back on the floor and bring the soles of your feet together so your knees bend outwards. You can choose to support your legs with a couple of cushions if that feels better for you. Allow your arms to rest on the floor, with your palms facing upwards. This position opens up your lungs and puts you in the perfect place to try some relaxing breathing.

Child's Pose
Kneel on the floor and bend down, stretching your arms out in front of you on the ground until your forehead touches the floor. Don't worry if your forehead doesn't quite reach, you can just put a cushion or bolster in front of you to rest on instead. After all, this is about relaxing, not over-stretching yourself.

Legs Up The Wall
Sit on the floor right next to a wall and manoeuvre yourself around until you're lying flat on your back with your legs straight up the wall. This is an inversion, which allows lots of blood to reach your head. You can also put a cushion under your hips if that's more comfortable for you.

Corpse Pose
The name might sound a bit sinister, but this pose is really soothing. And it's so easy to do, too. You simply lie flat on your back – with a cushion under your knees if you like – and your arms next to you with your palms facing up. If you want to feel even more relaxed, try to imagine you're lying in the sunshine and the sun's rays are warming your hands.

My Migraines
Fiona, 33

'I've been getting migraines since I was 16 years old and I know that stress and anxiety are triggers for me.

'Tiredness can contribute to my migraines, too, as I don't always sleep particularly well, and a friend recommended the Headspace meditation and mindfulness app to help me sleep. I found that I slept better when I used it, and over time if I kept up the habit I could better manage my stress levels, which reduced some of my migraines.

'At the same time my mother-in-law, who's a vicar, talked to me about her regular retreats to reflect and I did a bit of searching to see if I could find a retreat house in London where I could go to get some calm and quiet, to reflect and 'be not do'. For the last 18 months I've been attending the Open Reflective Days at the Royal Foundation of St Katharine about once every 3-4 months, and I've found that this time has been perfect for some quiet, soul-calming meditation and mindfulness, which helps to get me back on track.

'I also like to wander up to my local park and just sit in one of the gardens there and let my mind wander. The peace combined with an environment that is good for migraines is excellent.'

Chapter Nine

YOUR SENSES

*'Strong chemical smells, perfume, fluorescent lights and loud noises
can all be migraine triggers for me. I hate the supermarket aisles where
cleaning products are kept because of it!'*

Patsy, 64

Have you ever felt like you must have the nose of a Bloodhound or super hearing like Superman, because your senses are so much more sensitive than other people's? That's because of your migraines. Certain types of sensory stimulation, such as bright sunlight or the smell of strong coffee, can actually be triggers for migraines.

Sensory triggers can be tricky to handle, but it's easier when you know how. Of course, you're taking migraine management to a whole different level when you're faced with trying to avoid bright sunlight or the smell of someone else's perfume. Still, that doesn't mean that you have to sit back and let your migraines happen. There are things that you can do to keep your senses – and your head – happy.

Sights

You might already know that when you have a migraine you can get more sensitive to light or you may prefer to lie in a dark room. This is called photophobia, although it's more of an aversion to light than an actual fear of it. Migraines and photophobia go hand in hand around 80 per cent of the time. So if you have it, you're not alone.

As well as being difficult to handle during a migraine, light – such as bright or flickering lights – can also be a trigger for some people. You can come across it at the most inconvenient times, too, like the glaring sun as you're driving home from work or the flickering overhead lighting at a shopping mall. If this is a trigger for you, it might take just seconds for this light to cause you discomfort.

Remember back in the sleep chapter when we talked about the blue light waves that can keep you awake at night? Well, when it comes to photophobia, those blue light waves which come out of screens are the ones that can cause the most trouble. If this is a real problem for you, you can get screen filters and special glasses which aren't too expensive. They do exactly what the name says, they filter out the blue light that's coming from your screen without changing the appearance of it. These filters are easy to find for most types of devices.

There are other simple – and free – things that you can do to help if light is a trigger, too. Use your migraine diary to figure out if there are certain brightly-lit places or screen-based activities that seem to act as triggers. Once you've pinpointed a problem, try little things, like changing the angle of your computer screen on your desk so the glare of the sun doesn't reflect off of it, or choosing to read by a lamp with a dim glow rather than having a bright overhead light beaming down on you. If you find that fluorescent lighting at work is difficult for you, ask if you can use a desk lamp instead. And yes, when the sun's blazing brightly overhead, put on your sunglasses and wear a hat with a brim to shade your eyes. It's all pretty basic stuff, really.

Stripes Can Make You See Stars

Researchers in the Netherlands and the US have found that simply looking at stripes might trigger a migraine in some people. They discovered an increase in a type of brain activity called gamma oscillations when the people involved in the study looked at stripes, which didn't happen when they were viewing fluffy clouds or pictures of nature scenes. Experts don't know why, but vertical stripes, like those you'd see on a radiator, seem to be worse than horizontal stripes, such as Venetian blinds hanging in a window.

Smells

It's pretty common for a very strong or unpleasant smell to make someone feel unwell or cause a headache. Even people who don't get migraines might need a lie down when they're exposed to a particularly potent pong, like the smell of paint thinner, for example. But for those of us who live with migraines, powerful smells can trigger an attack, too.

Just like aversion to light, scientists have a word for this one, and sensitivity to smell is called osmophobia. This strong sense of smell that you can get during an attack might also cause you to feel sick. And whether or not you're having a migraine, you're more likely to be sensitive to smells than someone who's never had a migraine.

So you've got a delicate nose, and you don't want to risk a migraine. How do you avoid odours when they're all around us? There are some times, like when you're at home alone, when you can control any scents that you use and keep any heavily perfumed products far away. But when it comes to other people, or other places, the issue of smell can get a bit ... personal. Your aunt might not feel too pleased if you ask her not to wear her favourite perfume when you visit, and your business partner might be a bit confused when you ask her to move your meeting to somewhere other than the local coffee shop. So, try explaining that it's nothing personal but you are very sensitive to smells – even those that most people love – and that you could be ill for days because of it.

Later on in the book, we'll chat through putting together a migraine survival kit and why you should take it with you wherever you go. If you're sensitive to smells, you could try keeping an aroma that you like in your kit, so you can sniff it whenever you need to block out a less pleasant pong. Peppermint oil could be one to try, as separate studies done by German and Iranian researchers found it was helpful with headaches and migraines. In fact, the German study concluded that putting peppermint oil on your forehead at the start of a headache worked as well as taking 1,000mg of acetaminophen.

Smells That Stink

Nose twitching? Some strong odours that might be triggering your migraines can include:

Perfume

Petrol

Cooking smells

Cigarette smoke

Air fresheners and scented candles

Flowers

Cleaning products

Aerosol sprays

Paint thinner

Coffee

Sounds

You know that dark room that lots of us who live with migraines lie down in during an attack? It's a quiet room, right? When you've got a migraine you're hardly going to put on your favourite Taylor Swift song and sing along at the top of your lungs. Instead you'll probably seek out silence. And chances are you like a bit of peace and quiet even when you aren't in the middle of an attack. A survey done by the National Headache Foundation in the US showed that 51 per cent of people who get migraines avoid concerts where there will be loud music.

According to the Migraine Relief Center, which is also in the US, about 75 per cent of people who live with migraines are sensitive to noise. Loud noise can trigger a migraine and it might also make you feel worse when you're mid-attack. This noise sensitivity is called phonophobia, and it can also be a warning symptom. So, if the sound of your children laughing suddenly makes you want to cover your ears, ask yourself if they're really being too loud, or if you might just have a migraine coming on. If it is a migraine, this is a good time to do something about it before it gets worse.

Shhhh! Tips for keeping things quiet

Stay Away From Loud Noises
It seems kind of obvious, doesn't it? But just because you know that, for example, the construction sounds that came from next door when your neighbour was having building work done triggered a migraine, it doesn't mean that you'll think to keep away from things like fireworks displays or action films at the cinema. They may be different sounds, but they're still loud enough to act as a trigger.

Get a Pair of Earplugs
They aren't expensive and they could be a lifesaver at the right moment. Keep a set in your migraine survival kit, too.

Soften Echoey Rooms at Home
Hard surfaces cause sound to reverberate, while softer things, like carpets, absorb sound. Now, you may not want to entirely redecorate, but adding accessories like curtains, rugs and soft furnishings all soften sound in your home.

Move Away From the Noise
That's not to say that you need to go as far as moving house, but if there's a noisy road outside, simply switching your bed to the opposite wall in your bedroom – or to another room in your house, if you can – may be helpful.

Touch

When it comes to your sense of touch, it's likely to be things like cold and heat, or drastic changes in the weather, that trigger migraines.

You might not have even realised that there was a storm brewing or a cold snap coming until a migraine hit, but lightning, high humidity and drops in air pressure are all things that could affect you. This is stating the obvious, but the weather is usually more unsettled when the seasons are changing so keep that in mind as the next months go by. Of course, keeping track in your diary is the best way to know which types of weather affect you.

How does knowing this actually help you? After all, unless you pack up and move to Spain, you're not going to be able to improve what's going on outside your front door. Yes, the weather is one of those triggers that can leave you feeling a little bit out of control, but don't let this get you downhearted. While it's true that you can't wave a magic wand to stop it from snowing or to keep the high winds from blowing, there are still things that you can do to protect yourself from an attack when conditions get bad. If the weather knocks you off your feet, then knowledge is your best defence. And technology helps a lot, too.

If you've got a smartphone, you've probably got a weather app, which will tell you when there's likely to be lightning nearby or if it's shaping up to be a blustery day. So make it a habit to check the weather every day, and look ahead to the next few days, too. This will help you to plan in advance and know if you need to be extra careful for a while. Or if you find that air pressure is an issue for you, try downloading a free barometer app, which will tell you what the barometric pressure is wherever you are. Then on the days when your app tells you the air pressure's low, that it's a bad day for migraine sufferers or that thunderstorms are looming overhead, take it easy. Do whatever it takes to keep your other triggers balanced because you know that your body's bound to be under some strain.

My Migraines
Karen, 34

'I've discovered that the cold is a trigger for me. I live in Cornwall and I had a surf lesson in cold water on my birthday. Afterwards, I had a migraine and I think it was the temperature difference between the warmth of the day and the cold sea that triggered it.

'When I get migraines, they start with tiredness and then I get an aura that causes my vision to become so blurry that eventually I can *only see things on the periphery. Then the headache starts around my eyes and feels like it's going right through my brain.*

'Drinking coffee or Coke can help. I've only ever taken paracetamol and ibuprofen for my migraines, but sometimes they don't even touch the sides. I just have to lie on the sofa with the curtains shut as I know it will last for two days. It's so debilitating, I feel like I'm in this bubbly atmosphere inside my head and I can't even get myself a drink of water.

'Thankfully, I don't have them as often as I used to. That's because I avoid red wine and dark chocolate, I wear sunglasses or a hat on sunny days and, of course, I can't go in the sea, not even when my son wants me to go in with him.'

Migraines at Work

According to the Migraine Trust, in the UK there are an estimated 25 million work and school days missed each year because of migraines. It can be pretty worrying when migraines affect you at work, and that extra stress isn't going to help you, either. Instead, it just might trigger more attacks, which would make the whole situation worse. But you don't have to tackle it alone, so although it might seem like a difficult thing to do, ask your boss or HR department for help.

'All employers have a duty of care to ensure their employees are provided with a safe, healthy and productive working environment,' says Sarah Sen, Director, Sen HR Consulting. 'Employers are expected to make reasonable adjustments for employees with long-term health conditions such as migraine. As a minimum, employers should consider identifying and tackling workplace stress, recognising and managing migraine triggers at work and consider flexible working options to enable the sufferer to work around their disability where appropriate.'

Your employer will have sickness policies and procedures, although, because of your disorder, you may find that you need to take more time off than most people. But Sarah says that there should also be a framework in place for supporting employees with long-term health issues.

You might find that you're getting migraines because you're being bombarded with triggers at work. If you're finding this difficult, speak to someone about it who can help you. Remember that your employer wants you at work, not off sick. So if the overhead lighting or the smell of food being heated up is affecting you, talk about what can be done to change things for the better. It may be something as simple as moving you to an area of your workplace that's further away from the kitchen, for example.

'Employees suffering with migraine are encouraged to tell their employer as soon as possible so that they are able to provide support and understand how the condition affects them,' explains Sarah. 'Whilst it can seem like a daunting thing to do, most employers will appreciate an employee's honesty and will work with them to identify and address any workplace triggers.'

So the sooner you speak to someone at work about your migraines, the sooner they can help you out, whether that means creating a more flexible working arrangement for you or simply helping to reduce your triggers at work. Your employer might also ask for permission to speak to your GP or specialist, which could help them to get a better understanding of your migraines and provide better support for you.

My Migraines
Patsy, 64

> 'I was so young when I started getting migraines that I can't remember not having them.
>
> 'Strong chemical smells, fluorescent lights and thundery, humid weather can all be triggers for me, among other things.
>
> 'Having these sorts of triggers means that I have to be careful wherever I go. When I was younger I had to wear ear plugs to discos and as soon as any strobe lighting started flickering, I had to get off the dance floor. Even then, nine times out of 10, I'd get a migraine anyway so I stopped going to discos altogether.
>
> 'These days, a trip to the supermarket can trigger a migraine if I'm not careful. I'm particularly sensitive to fluorescent lights and I can see them flickering when nobody else can. Plus, the smells in the aisles where soap powders and other chemical-based products are stocked is too overpowering for me. So I wear my sunglasses to protect myself from the lights and I avoid certain aisles, too – my husband shops for cleaning products so I don't have to. It makes a real difference, even though I feel a bit stupid wearing sunglasses indoors!'

Chapter Ten

YOUR MIGRAINE DIARY

'It's only with committing to a proper diary and looking for patterns that you can see what's triggering migraines.'

Dr Mike Unwin, GP

You've probably already worked out that your migraine diary is one of the most important tools that you can use to take charge of your migraines. Why? Because your migraines are unique and keeping a diary of your attacks helps you to spot the patterns which will show you what's triggering them. For example, your diary might reveal that your warning symptoms always seem to come on at the same time of day or in the same place. Or maybe it happens after you've been on a big night out which has interfered with your sleep patterns, or when you've been running late and have skipped a meal. Think of it as solving a mystery, and your migraine diary is where you'll find the clues you need to understand what your own personal triggers are.

Of course, when you're in the throes of an attack, it can be hard to see or think straight, let alone put pen to paper and write down how you're feeling. So don't feel like you have to put yourself under any pressure to take notes as it's happening. Be kind to yourself when you're not feeling well and once things improve, fill in your diary while it's still fresh in your mind. By keeping note of your migraines when you can and reviewing what you've been through once you have a clear head, you'll begin to learn how you can change the little things in your life which can make a big difference, like drinking more water every day or carrying your sunglasses with you at all times.

Nobody wants you to have migraines, so please don't encourage them to come on just to have something to write down! That would be madness. It also means that your diary wouldn't be a true record of your usual lifestyle, which is what we're aiming for here. You need to spot those sneaky triggers in your normal day that might not be so obvious. So instead have your diary handy for when you might need it and go about your days – and nights – as normal.

Now, once you've started using your diary you may spot a trigger straight away and realise what changes you can make, which would be fantastic. You may also have to wait until you've had a few migraines in order to identify a common theme. Of course, that's not ideal, and the point of this exercise is for you to suffer less. But the fact is, these migraines are going to happen whether or not you fill out a diary about them. As frustrating as that is, you might as well use them to get some ammunition in order to fight back and find your balance.

It's actually a good idea to keep a migraine diary for a few months and record the details of every migraine you have in that time in order to truly spot patterns in your migraines – or your lifestyle – that can help. Over these months, if you discover a trigger, try making the lifestyle changes to avoid it, but carry on with the diary. Then you can keep track of the positive effect that say, getting up at the same time each morning, or avoiding alcohol actually has on your migraines. And if it doesn't help, you'll be able to look back at your diary again to try and see if there was a different trigger at play all along.

'Don't pull the tiger's tail,' says Dr Goadsby. 'If you do, and it bites you, don't complain.' In other words, once you've worked out that something triggers your migraines, avoid it. It's very easy to slip back into old habits and have a lie in or be tempted to have a cup of coffee after dinner even though you know it can be a trigger for you, because it's nice, right? But it seems crazy to go to all the effort of using your diary to figure out what your triggers are only to ignore the results.

The other useful thing about having a migraine diary is that you can take it to your GP or headache specialist and use it to show them exactly what you've been going through. Doctors can only help you if they've got all of the details. Going in to your GP and saying that you have a lot of migraines is too vague for them to be able to understand just what you're going through and how migraines affect you. If you take your diary, however, they'll be able to see just how severe and disabling your attacks are and will be able to use it to work with you in order to offer you the treatment you need.

The diary over the page is a guide that you can use, but it's not prescriptive by any means. If you like it, photocopy it, draw it out by hand, take a photo on your phone ... do whatever you need to do so that you can use it to keep a record of your migraines. If you'd rather keep track of your migraines in a diary that you already keep online, or take down notes on your mobile, then do that instead. There are also migraine diary apps that you can download onto your phone, like Migraine Buddy, which can help you to keep track, too.

It doesn't matter what method you choose, the important thing is that you start – today. Make things easy for yourself and have your phone, diary or photocopied sheets ready so that when a migraine hits and you need to take those important notes, you're not scrabbling to download an app or make photocopies. Plus, having your diary ready means that you'll be able to jot things down while they're still fresh in your mind, which is when they're most accurate. And remember to write as much as you can in each section. The more information you collect, the more you'll understand about what's going on in your body.

Then, you'll be on your way towards taking control of your migraines.

Migraine Diary Sheet

Date and time your migraine started:

Date and time your migraine finished:

How long did it last?

Warning Phase Symptoms:

Aura Symptoms:

Attack Phase Symptoms:

Resolution Phase Symptoms:

Recovery Phase Symptoms:

Triggers
List any possible triggers for this migraine

Treatment
Any Medication Taken:

Did you do anything else to help relieve your migraine?

What helped?

What didn't?

PART THREE

OTHER THINGS YOU CAN DO

'Be sensible and don't go out without your medicines.'
Peter J. Goadsby, Director NIHR/Wellcome Trust King's Clinical Research
Facility and Professor of Neurology, King's College London

Chapter Eleven

HOW YOUR DOCTOR CAN HELP

'Since starting Botox for my chronic migraines, I still get them but not half as often. Plus I only get the zigzag aura and no pain. It's amazing.'

Rhian, 31

Not everyone who gets migraines will have been to a doctor for help. That's one of the reasons why only 50 per cent of migraine sufferers have been diagnosed. So you may very well be managing your attacks on your own, or you might have always followed your mum's advice based on what's worked for her. Or, maybe you have been to see your GP and are under the care of a headache centre.

Whatever your approach has been so far, it's worth knowing how your doctor can help and, if you do decide to ask for support, how to get the most help from your GP for your migraines. Then, when you're armed with the right information, you can make a decision about what to do next.

'If someone has been diagnosed with migraines, I'd ask about their diet and what's triggered the migraines,' says GP Dr Mike Unwin. 'Then I would find out how severe they were and how long the migraines lasted. It helps me to work out the treatment and see if it's worth taking preventative medication.'

Take Your Migraine Diary With You

Whatever you've got – your diary with your migraines noted in it, photocopies of the migraine diary sheet from this book, or an app that you've been using to record your migraines – remember to take it along and show your doctor exactly what you've been going through. In order to formally diagnose migraines your GP will probably ask you to fill in a migraine diary anyway and it will also help him to decide what treatment might be right for you.

He should also ask you some questions to make sure that there isn't something more serious causing you to feel unwell, just in case. But what he'll do with this information can vary.

'There are no set rules for referrals,' says Professor Goadsby. 'If you talk about your disability and what you can't do, you'll get more help from your GP than if you talk about suffering.'

So if you tell him that your migraines are making you sick, or they're extremely painful, chances are your GP will work to find solutions for these problems alone. However, painkillers and anti-sickness medications might only scratch the surface of the problem. If you tell your GP about all the days you've had to take off work, the times you've been lying in a dark room while someone else looked after your children, or when you missed out on day trips on holiday ... then you'll be more likely to get help for your migraines as a whole. This is because a GP tries to help with whatever you tell them, so it's up to you to give him the whole picture, particularly if your migraines are very disabling.

'It's the disability which matters,' explains Professor Goadsby. 'It costs the community.'

What the NHS Offers

Exactly what you might be offered on the NHS for your migraines depends on what symptoms you have, how often you get migraines and how severe they can be. That's why it's so important to go armed with all of the information you can for your GP, so you can get help tailored to your experience of migraines.

Here are some of the things you may be able to get on the NHS to help, depending on your individual needs:

- **Medication**

  There are different types of medications available on the NHS to help with migraines. A commonly-used one is a type of drug called triptans, which help to reduce pain messages and narrow blood vessels in your head. Other medications that you might get offered include anti-sickness medication and painkillers. There's more information about these in the next chapter, but keep in mind that the treatment that will work for you is as individual as your migraines themselves. Your doctor can help you to figure out which you could try, but it can be a matter of trial and error to find out what works for you. So carry on using your diary while you're trying any new medication and keep track of what's working – and what isn't. If you need to, go back to your doctor and ask whether it's time to try something different.

If you're getting migraines very frequently, you might be offered medication to prevent them. This could be beta blockers, or you could be given something like anti-depressants, or medication that's usually used for epilepsy. There is also a new preventative medication just for migraines called Aimovig, which is available in the US and will hopefully be approved in the UK soon. Keep in mind that it can take a few months for preventative medication to work, so don't give up on it if your migraines don't disappear as soon as you start taking it. You might just need a bit more time.

If you get a prescription, your GP will choose a drug that will suit you. The sorts of things that she'll think about when deciding what to give you are the type of migraines you get, whether you're likely to become pregnant and whether you're taking any sort of contraception.

On the Migraine Trust Charity's website (www.migrainetrust.org) you'll find a long list of painkillers, anti-sickness drugs and drugs given for the prevention and treatment of migraines, rather than just the symptoms. Some are tablets, some dissolve on the tongue, some are available at the chemist and some need a prescription. You may find that the treatment that works for you is completely different from the one that helps a friend, or even your brother. Sometimes, it's just a matter of trial and error, and, of course, not every medication will be suitable for every person.

If you've been taking a migraine medication for a while and you feel like it isn't working as well as it used to, work with your doctor to figure out your best plan of action. Don't forget to take your diary with you to show him or her what you've tried in the past, and how effective it was for you.

- **Referral**

  If your GP feels that it's necessary for you to get some extra help, you can get a referral to a GP with a special interest in headache or a neurologist. Some of the treatments that you'll read about below, like TMS and Botox, can be offered by your specialist once you've been referred.

- **Botox**

  Botox – yes, the beauty treatment injections that you can have done to relax the muscles in your face and keep you looking wrinkle-free – is also used for people with chronic migraines on the NHS. Experts think that Botox may work for migraines by interrupting nerve signals in your brain. It won't suit everyone, and it has to be done by a specialist, but it may help to reduce the number of attacks that you get. If you had Botox for migraines, you'd usually have treatment every 12 weeks and, if it's going to work for you, you'd know within 24 weeks.

- **Acupuncture**

  Acupuncture is a very old form of Chinese medicine. In Chinese medicine, there's a belief that there's something called qi (pronounced 'chi'), which is a life force that flows through the body at all times. And if you are unwell, your qi is disturbed and needs attention. When you have acupuncture, the treatment restores the proper flow of qi throughout your body. It's a very different way of thinking to what we're used to with Western medicine, but it can have good results.

  A study that was done in China found that when people who lived with migraines with aura were given acupuncture, they had fewer attacks. Even when they did have migraines, the attacks were less severe and didn't last as long as they used to.

  When you have the treatment, you'll either lie down or sit up and your acupuncturist will place very small, fine, sterile needles into your skin on certain spots on the body called acupuncture points.

  If you're lucky, you may be able to get up to 10 sessions of acupuncture for migraines on the NHS, but unfortunately, in many areas, it simply isn't available. If you do have acupuncture on the NHS, it's probably going to be done by your GP or a physiotherapist.

My Migraines
Rhian, 31

> 'I suffer with chronic migraines. They start with a tiny spot in my vision, which turns into a zigzag effect in both eyes, then I lose my vision completely apart from the zigzags. After that, I get sick – so very sick – and my head feels like it's going to explode.
>
> 'Since starting Botox last year, my life has changed. I have 32 injections every 12 weeks and now I don't have half as many migraines as I used to. When I do have a migraine, I still get the zigzags but not the pain. And as the severe pain was what had caused me to be sick, I don't vomit anymore either. The visual disturbance might last for half an hour and then it's gone. Once it passes I can get on with my life!'

Chapter Twelve

WHEN ALL ELSE FAILS

'I find that when I get a migraine, the best thing that I can do to make it go away is go to sleep. But if it's a bad one, I've got painkillers that I can take, too. I decide which ones to take depending on how severe it is.'

Janet, 78

It would be fantastic to be able to tell you that, if you follow all of the advice in this book, you'll never have to live with another migraine again. Only here's the thing about migraines – they're sneaky little monsters. Even when you've done all of your reading, when you've listened to your body, completed your diary and made lifestyle choices to eliminate triggers, the odd migraine can still slip past your defences. Because although you're doing everything that you can to create the balance that you need, life can be unpredictable sometimes. Plus, over time, life changes, and your body changes. Your migraines and your triggers can change, too.

So, as well as being armed with a firm understanding of your own migraines, it's important to have some migraine treatment information at your fingertips. Just in case. And if you never have to use it, well, that would be even better, wouldn't it?

Show Denial The Door

In the course of interviewing people for this book, when they talked about their warning symptoms, one thing came up again and again. And generally it was, 'No, not another migraine, it can't be'. You might be able to relate to that. From time to time you might have convinced yourself that you were feeling completely drained just because you hadn't been sleeping very well, or that the reason you'd just inhaled a massive Dairy Milk bar was because you had PMT. Because anything would be better than admitting that you're getting yet another migraine, right? But then it's only when your eyes cloud over with an aura or the pain hits like a jackhammer in your brain that you finally accept what's really happening. And let's face it, by then you probably feel so ill that you have no choice but to surrender your stubbornness and admit that you're having a migraine.

'Don't let perfection be the enemy of good,' says Professor Goadsby. That's good advice. While giving in to a migraine is never a nice feeling, being in denial of your warning symptoms really won't help you get through this attack. In fact, you could wind up feeling much worse because of it. Denying that a migraine is on its way won't get you the anti-nausea medication, the pain relief, the big glass of water or the rest that could ease your symptoms. And it won't make your migraine stop, either, because – as anyone who lives with migraines knows – that train will just keep on coming, whether you want to board it or not. So when you feel like your body just might be warning you that a migraine is on its way, take it seriously. And if it does turn out to be simple tiredness or plain old PMT, then, hooray, you didn't get a migraine! If not, you've given yourself a chance to get some help before things get even more intense. Or you might even stop it altogether. And isn't that better than pretending it's not happening at all?

Plan Your Migraines

Yes, you read that right. And no, that doesn't mean that you shouldn't try to prevent migraines. What it means is that if you know that you can be at risk of the occasional attack, you don't want them to happen at the most inconvenient time, do you? Instead you can make choices so those attacks happen at a time that's best for you.

Of course, you'll never have a day in your diary with the word MIGRAINE written in it, as if it were a date or a dentist's appointment. There's never a good day to spend in pain or vomiting for hours on end. But when you know what your triggers are, you can decide whether or not to expose yourself to them and risk getting a migraine. And if you've got something coming up in your life that is bound to lead to an attack, you can decide when the best day would be to do it, or how to minimise attacks during the time around that day so that you don't get completely pummelled by them.

For example, maybe you have a strict 10pm bedtime in order to keep migraines at bay, but next month you're going to be a bridesmaid at your sister's wedding and you know you'll be up late that night. Or perhaps you're going on holiday and you know you'll have to cope with jet lag. Spotting triggers before they happen means you that can minimise the effects, and even schedule in some time for them. Professor Goadsby suggests that you can plan your life so that if you do wind up having the occasional migraine, they happen on the days that suit you, not the days when you need to be at your best.

Let's say that you're dying to take that jet lag-riddled holiday, but you're frightened that migraines will ruin the whole thing. What you need to do is think ahead and plan to be kind to yourself. One way of doing this would be to build in an extra day or two into your holiday – or plan for an easy couple of days at either end – in order to accommodate for the jet lag. Also, drinking lots of water on the plane, avoiding alcohol or any food that may trigger your migraines and sleeping when you need to so that you can adjust to the new time zone can all help too.

How about your sister's wedding? It can be a bit worrying if someone else is planning an event that doesn't fit in with the lifestyle choices that you make in order to prevent attacks, but there are things that you can do to protect yourself. First of all, do everything in your power to stay migraine-free in the days or weeks leading up to the wedding – and, of course, on the day itself. Chances are, it will be an unusually busy day and your mealtimes won't be consistent, so plan to eat regularly and have a bottle of water to hand so you can keep sipping from it throughout the day to stay hydrated. It won't detract from the bride's day if you sneak out to nibble on a sandwich after you get your hair done, right? In fact, it would be better for you to do that than to disappear in agony just before the ceremony. And, if you really need to, once you've celebrated with the happy couple, slip off for a slightly earlier night to get an extra hour in bed.

So if you know that you're going to have the odd migraine, then do whatever you can to limit their impact as much as possible. Not only will you suffer less, but you'll feel more in control of your disorder.

Ways to Ease a Migraine

- **Medication**

  In the previous chapter, we talked about what sort of drugs you might get on the NHS to treat your migraines, and, chances are, you've already tried some medication to ease your attacks. Maybe you've only ever had over the counter painkillers or maybe you're already taking a prescription the doctor's given you for your migraines. Either way, if what you've got works, stick with it. If not, it might be a good idea to look into getting something different so you've got it ready to try, just in case you need it.

When you have a migraine, your digestive system slows down, so when it comes to painkillers, soluble or fast-acting drugs which are absorbed more quickly might be worth a try. Then you don't have to rely as much on your sluggish digestion to bring you relief.

The prescription medications available, like triptans, don't work for everyone, but the only way to know which ones might be any good for you is to chat to your doctor about it and then give the one that he suggests a go the next time you have an attack.

Also, keep in mind that if you get sick during migraines, you may get better results from injections, nasal sprays, or even suppositories instead of tablets that you have to swallow. After all, tablets aren't of much use if you've brought them back up again.

Finally, when it comes to migraine medication and painkillers, please be careful. It's understandable that when the searing pain of a migraine hits, you just want it to go away – fast. But sometimes people who have migraines take painkillers or triptans so often that they wind up getting medication overuse headaches, which you might also have heard of as a rebound headache. These headaches are different to migraine, though, because they're dull headaches that you get every day, which might feel worse in the morning. If you have rebound headaches, you'll need to stop taking the drugs that are causing it, although instead of going cold turkey it would be better to taper them off under the guidance of your doctor.

- **Eat and Drink if You Can**

Don't worry, this isn't going to be a mini-lecture on how to stick to your healthy diet mid-migraine. Of course, while it's never ideal to let your blood sugar levels go crazy, the truth is that when you have a migraine you're probably just going to do whatever you can to get through it. It's pretty hard to argue with that. So while you might avoid coffee most of the time, it can be a great idea to grab a strong cup of the stuff when you start to feel woozy to let the caffeine work its magic. If that does the trick for you, then go for it.

It's tricky enough to manage an attack at the best of times and it's not going to help you to add more stress by trying to stick to a super-healthy diet when you're feeling at your worst. Also, don't forget that during the warning phase of your migraines you might get cravings. So don't be hard on yourself if you wind up eating chocolate or chips just to cope. But once you're through to the other side, try to get your diet back on track so you don't trigger another attack, OK?

That said, if you're feeling queasy or being sick, food will probably be the last thing on your mind, but getting dehydrated won't help you, either; try to nibble on bits of bland food, like toast or clear soup, and take small sips of water, too. You might even find that drinking water when a migraine starts can ease your symptoms.

When you have a migraine, it's usually a good idea to avoid strong-smelling food, especially if you get sick. But trust your instincts and if you feel like eating something, do. Some people who were interviewed for this book said they find that certain sensations in their mouth – like chewing gum or sucking on boiled sweets – can ease the crushing jaw pain that they get during a migraine, as well. And if you do feel like eating, give something with ginger in it a try. One study done in Iran found that 250mg of ginger powder can be nearly as effective as 50mg of the drug Sumitriptan at relieving migraines. Ginger can be good for staving off nausea, too.

As the worst of your migraine shifts, you might feel that fierce recovery phase hunger taking over. This can be a nice time to get some healthy food inside you, and to start to find your balance again.

- **Dress the Part**

  It's a safe bet that while you're curled up in a dark room wishing your migraine away, what you look like and what you're wearing are going to be the last things on your mind. Still, it's a good idea to think about what you've got on. Wearing something that's loose around your waist can help you with any nausea or stomach trouble that might be making you uncomfortable. And if you find it difficult to tolerate sunlight or fluorescent lights, try wearing sunglasses, even if you're indoors.

- **Sleep, or At Least Rest**

  Although too much sleep can be a trigger for some people, getting some shut-eye at the right time can work wonders during an attack. You might even find that your body is crying out for sleep and that you haven't got much choice in the matter.

  'The ideal thing would be to shut the curtains, have a rest and sleep it off,' says Dr Ahmed. 'But sometimes it's not possible for mums with young children or people who are at work, so take the appropriate medication and do as little as you can.'

  If you find it difficult to sleep when you've got a migraine, don't give up on resting. Simply lying still can help, too. This is because moving around – particularly moving your head – might make your symptoms feel worse.

At the very least, take things very slowly and try not to make any sudden head movements.

- **Go Easy on Your Senses**

  When you're having a migraine, you might find that you instinctively choose to rest in a quiet, dark room. Remember that an attack might make you sensitive to light, sound, smells and touch, so find yourself some peace. Stay away from screens as much as you can and if daylight and background noise can get too much for you, try blocking it all out with an eye mask and earplugs. Use a pleasant smell, like the scent of peppermint oil, to block out any smells that are unbearable when your nose is particularly sensitive and, although this might sound obvious, if something makes your skin hurt, don't do it. Nobody's going to care if you're lying in bed with unbrushed hair because your scalp can't stand the sensation.

- **Change Your Plans**

  Or better yet, cancel them. Sometimes your migraines might be so powerful that you'll have no choice, and you probably won't want to go out during a severe attack, either. However, if you're in the early stages of a migraine – or are simply having a milder attack – you might be tempted to push yourself to carry on as you normally would. Yes, it can be frustrating and disappointing to have to cancel your plans when you have a migraine, particularly if you wind up doing this over and over again. But it doesn't matter how severe your migraine is, going out to the cinema or meeting friends for lunch simply isn't going to help. And chances are you won't enjoy yourself as much as you usually would, and you won't be great company, either. Even when the attack phase has finished and you're starting to feel better, remember that your migraine isn't over until after the resolution phase has finished, and you still won't be at your best because during that time you might feel woozy and tired, among other things. So listen to your body, give yourself a break, and reschedule whatever plans you need to.

- **Have a Cold Shower**

  Or a hot one, if that's what works for you. Just remember not to turn the temperature up too much! Getting scalded in a super-hot shower won't make things better. You could also try a hot water bottle, a heated wheat bag, or a cold flannel or an ice pack wrapped in a towel on your forehead or the back of your neck.

How To Create A Migraine Survival Kit

Once you've used your migraine diary to get a better understanding of what eases your attacks, use that information to put together a migraine survival kit – and keep it with you at all times. Because let's face it, when that sickness starts swelling up in your stomach, you don't want to be scrabbling around at the back of the bathroom cabinet for anti-nausea tablets. The point is to have your treatments to hand, whenever you might need them, so you can grab them without having to think twice about it.

That might mean keeping some medication, a bottle of water and a can of cola in your handbag or desk drawer. Or, if you don't want to lug everything around with you, put a few survival kits together to keep at home, at work and in the car, just in case. And keep another one by your bed that also contains an eye mask, some earplugs and a hot water bottle or flannel. Then you can relax, knowing that if a migraine does strike, you're covered.

What to Put in Your Migraine Survival Kit

Of course, ideally, once you've worked out what your triggers are, you won't need your migraine survival kit. Or at least you won't need it as often as you used to. Still, having one close by is a great insurance policy in case you do have to use it at some point. This list is just an idea of some of the things that you can have in your kit, you can leave out whatever isn't useful to you and include something else that you find helpful. What matters is that you have one that suits you.

If you do get an attack and wind up using something from your kit, don't forget to replenish the bits you've taken out of it once you're feeling better. After all, a kit full of empty boxes isn't going to help anyone.

Your migraine survival kit could include:

- A bottle of water
- A can of cola
- Your prescription medication
- Painkillers that work for you
- Peppermint oil if you find that the scent helps when you're exposed to strong smells
- Sunglasses and/or a wide-brimmed hat if you're sensitive to light
- A flannel, ice pack, wheat bag or hot water bottle, depending on what works for you
- A migraine diary sheet and pen so you can record what's happening

---

Quick Response

'The medicines we have work better the earlier you take them,' says Professor Goadsby. 'It won't help if you're throwing them up.'

Those are very wise words. Plus, once you spot your warning signals, you want to make sure that you take the pain relief that you need in time for it to get into your bloodstream before the worst of the pain hits. That's why it's so important to take your warning symptoms seriously and always carry your survival kit with you, or at least keep one nearby at all times. Because even with the best intentions, you never know where you might be when you'll start to feel spaced out or begin craving sweets. And by the time you've managed to drag yourself to the closest pharmacy for some painkillers, you may have already been walloped by the full force of your migraine. It's much, much better to hit your migraine before it hits you.

Should You Ever Go to Hospital With a Migraine?

It's pretty scary to think that your migraines could ever be so severe that you'd need to go to hospital. Rest assured that, generally, your migraines won't be doing you any harm, even if it does feel like there's an actual drill going through your brain. That said, there are other health conditions which can feel similar to a migraine and can be pretty serious. So, if your migraine feels extreme in any way – if the pain is far more severe than normal, if you can't stop being sick, if you fall unconscious, if the pain has come on very suddenly, if you experience sudden weakness, or if you have trouble speaking or walking – you need to call 999 or go to A&E.

If you're not sure about whether your super-severe migraine is an emergency or not, at the very least call 111, the NHS non-emergency number, for advice. Or get someone to phone them for you if you're in too much pain or are finding it too difficult to speak properly. It might just be that you are having a particularly unbearable migraine. But it would be much worse to have a serious condition go untreated than it would to ask for help and be told that you're having a severe migraine. And remember, if you do end up in hospital with a whopper of an attack, the doctors may be able to help you with your symptoms. At that stage, any help can be a welcome relief.

My Migraines
Janet, 78

> *'When I get a migraine, it's usually an aura that looks like flashing lights in front of my eyes, and a headache. But sometimes I get nausea,*

too. My worst one started when I was in a car behind a lorry on the motorway and the exhaust fumes triggered a migraine. By the time I got home I was vomiting and had diarrhoea. I crawled up to bed and just stayed there until I could move again.

'What I do to treat my migraines depends on how it feels. If the pain isn't too bad, I can sometimes get away with taking over the counter painkillers. But if it's more severe and I feel sick, I'll take a soluble painkiller that my doctor gave me called diclofenac. With other migraines, I just get the flashing lights of an aura. Then I can go to sleep and I'll be OK.'

Once You're Feeling Better

Once a migraine has passed and you finally feel like yourself again, you might want to forget all about it and just get on with your life. But this is actually a good time to go back to the beginning and work out what just happened. If you have been doing everything that's right for you, and you find your migraines are getting more frequent or more powerful, get that all-important diary out again. Have a think about whether you've had a change in routine, like maybe a new job or a change in your diet. Perhaps you haven't been getting much exercise lately, or maybe there are some hormonal changes going on that you hadn't even realised were happening. Stop and think about whether your sleep's been affected or if you might have developed a trigger that's completely new to you. Keep your mind open, speak to your doctor, take stock of what's going on in your life and what's happening in your body. And see your specialist if you need to.

Then use all of that help and information to take charge of your migraines and find your balance again. Because, let's face it, migraines are pretty powerful, and they can have a huge impact on every part of your life. Even if you had things perfectly balanced for a while, simply having an attack can throw you way off kilter. But it doesn't have to stay that way. You can find your balance and you can feel well again.

Just because you have this disorder, doesn't mean that you should have to suffer.

FOR MORE INFORMATION

Sleep
Rachel McGuinness, Sleep Coach
www.wakeupwithzest.com

Nutrition
Claudine Mules, Registered Nutritional Therapist
www.nutrivite.co.uk

Yoga
Pauline Gibbons, Tring Yoga Studio
www.tringyogastudio.uk

Mindfulness
Dr Lisa Greenspan, Chartered Counselling Psychologist
www.lisagreenspantherapy.com

Useful Apps
Daily Water
Migraine Buddy
Headspace

Migraine Charities
The Migraine Trust – www.migrainetrust.org
Migraine Action – www.migraine.org.uk